José Francis de Oliveira

Perinatal Fluoxetine-induced Neurofunctional Changes

José Francis de Oliveira

Perinatal Fluoxetine-induced Neurofunctional Changes

Animal Model Study

ScienciaScripts

Imprint
Any brand names and product names mentioned in this book are subject to trademark, brand or patent protection and are trademarks or registered trademarks of their respective holders. The use of brand names, product names, common names, trade names, product descriptions etc. even without a particular marking in this work is in no way to be construed to mean that such names may be regarded as unrestricted in respect of trademark and brand protection legislation and could thus be used by anyone.

Cover image: www.ingimage.com

This book is a translation from the original published under ISBN 978-620-2-17907-2.

Publisher:
Sciencia Scripts
is a trademark of
Dodo Books Indian Ocean Ltd. and OmniScriptum S.R.L publishing group

120 High Road, East Finchley, London, N2 9ED, United Kingdom
Str. Armeneasca 28/1, office 1, Chisinau MD-2012, Republic of Moldova, Europe
Printed at: see last page
ISBN: 978-620-7-21235-4

CONTENTS

CHAPTER 1

Depression is a highly prevalent psychiatric disorder and is associated with high levels of morbidity and mortality[1] . During pregnancy and breastfeeding, 10% of women may experience depression[2] , and pharmacological treatment during this period is recommended, despite the potential undesirable effects on the foetus, for two main reasons: [1] previous studies have shown that most antidepressant drugs do not cause morphological changes[3, 4] , and [2] the benefits of pharmacological treatment outweigh the potential risks to the developing foetus/neonate. For these reasons, it is estimated that 2 to 3% of pregnant women will use antidepressant drugs, of which selective serotonin reuptake inhibitors (SSRIs) are the most commonly used[5] . However, few studies have carried out a continuous assessment of children who were exposed to SSRIs during pregnancy and/or breastfeeding to examine whether this exposure could affect the individual's psychological and cognitive development.

Fluoxetine (FLX) is an SSRI and, as such, acts by blocking the reuptake of serotonin (5-HT) in the synaptic cleft, consequently increasing the bioavailability of this neurotransmitter[6] . FLX has been widely prescribed for the treatment of mood disorders due to its therapeutic efficacy and few side effects compared to other antidepressants[7] . This drug crosses the placental barrier in humans and rodents[8, 9] and is excreted in milk[10-12] , as well as inhibiting multidrug efflux proteins, such as phosphoglycoprotein P (PgP), which is present in the placental barrier[13] . Therefore, the use of FLX during pregnancy exposes the foetus to high levels of 5-HT as well as potential xenobiotics and/or other physiological molecules, such as glucocorticoids, which under normal conditions would be blocked in the placenta by PgP, which could lead to changes in the circulating levels of these molecules in the foetus and possible alterations in its development.

5-HT is a key regulator of various neurodevelopmental processes, such as cell migration, axonal growth, long-term potentiation, synaptogenesis, neural circuit formation and neurogenesis[14-18]. In addition, the formation of the raphe nuclei, which are the main serotonergic nuclei in the encephalon, is a complex, multi-stage process, subject to alterations by various substances that may come into contact with the foetus during its formation[19]. Studies have shown that 5-HT influences the development of the Central Nervous System from its earliest ontogeny; even when the foetus is still unable to synthesise 5-HT, serotonergic receptors are already present in the forming cerebral cortex, and the placenta produces and supplies the foetus with 5-HT during this period, until the formation of the raphe nuclei is complete and the foetus begins to produce its own 5-HT[20].

Disturbances in serotonergic signalling, even during strict periods of pre- and post-natal development, can result in long-term behavioural abnormalities[21-24] or predispose the individual to develop neuropsychiatric disorders during adulthood, such as anxiety, autism and depression[21-27]. This is believed to occur through alterations in the serotonergic modulation of important processes during neurodevelopment, such as the formation of neural circuits and synaptogenesis. Another hypothesis is based on possible neurotoxicity due to exposure of the developing nervous system to other molecules that would normally be prevented from reaching the foetus by the reverse transport carried out by placental PgP.

Studies with animals knocked out for the serotonin transporter (5-HTT) showed altered exploratory behaviour. These animals showed reduced horizontal exploration in the centre of the open field and normal exploration in the periphery, but reduced vertical exploration when compared to controls. The authors suggested that these effects could be associated with alterations in the somatosensory cortex, associated with tigmotaxis, since high levels of 5-HT during neurodevelopment impair the formation of this structure[28, 29]. 5-HTT knockout animals also show greater aversion to open and illuminated environments[30], and greater aversion to the central area in the open field test and to open arms in the elevated cross maze[31]. This evidence, added to the altered exploratory behaviour, leads to the conclusion that these animals show anxiety-like behaviour. Similar results have been found when 5-HTT is blocked by perinatal exposure to FLX[32]. An interesting fact that has been described is that only the blockade of 5-HTT leads to behavioural changes in later life; the blockade of the norepinephrine transporter (another neurotransmitter) did not cause the same change[33] .

There is a consensus that 5-HTT knockout animals, or those exposed to increased levels of 5-HT during development, also show behaviours similar to depression. Popa et al.[21] found increased immobility in the forced swim and tail suspension tests. Further corroborating this idea, animals deficient in 5-HT during development show a decrease in anxiety-like behaviours and an increase in aggression[34] . However, 5-HTT knockout mice do not show anhedonia[35] , which is one of the symptoms of depression, but 5-HTT knockout mice are anhedonic[31] . However, it is possible that these depression-like symptoms are the result of an inability of the serotonergic system to control the increased release of 5-HT induced by a stressful event, since the joint occurrence of stress during the perinatal period with reduced reuptake of 5-HT results in gene alterations in the serotonergic and stress systems, alterations which are associated with reduced ability to adapt to the environment in adulthood, as well as anxiety[36] . Since stress is one of the main factors involved in the development of depression, alterations in the brain's stress system due to exposure to high levels of 5-HT during development could increase susceptibility to the development of depression in later life.

Homberg et al[37] demonstrated that rodents knocked out for 5-HTT show an increase in cocaine-induced conditioned place preference; however, only knockout rats show an increase in cocaine self-administration, suggesting that, among rodents, rats are more sensitive to this psychotropic drug. These animals also show reduced social behaviour, as observed by the same author[38] in the social interaction test. In addition, other authors have also found a reduction in the aggressive behaviour of these animals[27, 39] .

In relation to cognitive abilities, Olivier et al[40] found results that led them to conclude that 5-HTT knockout animals show slight impairment in spatial and object memory, dependent on the hippocampus. This could be explained by probable differences in the serotonergic modulation of the neurodevelopment of the hippocampus and amygdala.

5-HT has been related to the stress response since its discovery, and this topic has been the focus of intense research ever since[41] . In addition, the hypothalamic-pituitary-adrenal (HPA) axis may be hyperactive in depression[42] . It is also known that maternal stress during pregnancy and breastfeeding, as well as stress during childhood and adolescence, results in sensitisation of the child's HPA axis, making their response to subsequent stressful events altered[43] . This ability of the maternal/infant environment to modify the basal activity of the HPA axis, as well as its response to stressful events in later life, was described 50 years ago, but only recently has this topic gained attention[44] . The realisation that events that occur during the development of the organism, such as maternal exposure to drugs, can have a late influence on the health of the individual has led to the development of a growing area of research called "*Developmental Origins of Health* and Disease" or DOHaD. The *DOHaD* paradigm is based on the influence of the environment in the early stages of foetal and postnatal development on the morphological and functional development of organs and its association with the origin of diseases later in life[45, 46] .

The neural system of stress comprises several areas, such as the amygdala and its subdivisions, the medial prefrontal cortex, the hippocampus, the bed nucleus of the stria terminalis (BNST) and the paraventricular nucleus (PVN). Each of these structures plays a different role in the response to a stressful event, which can be context-, gender- and age-dependent[47-49] . Furthermore, the stress system is of fundamental importance for survival, as it enables motor responses to avoid danger and allow escape, and through the formation of memory of past stressful events, the brain is able to programme future actions in subsequent contact with stressful events .[50]

Serotonergic receptors can modulate many of the brain structures involved in the stress response, and at least 14 subtypes of 5-HT receptors have been described, which couple to multiple intracellular signalling pathways, and we even have a serotonergic receptor that functions as a cation channel[51] . Therefore, changes in serotonergic tone during neurodevelopment in brain regions involved in the stress response can lead to changes in this response in adulthood[52] . It is important to emphasise that during adolescence, brain circuits are more sensitive to stressful events and are therefore more vulnerable to alterations that may become permanent in adulthood[53, 54]. However, deficiencies or abnormalities in the formation of neural circuits that can alter cognitive functions due to perinatal exposure to xenobiotics or drugs, such as CLX, can remain quiescent and only manifest themselves in the face of a challenge to brain function.[55]

Taken together, these data from the literature presented above provide evidence that alterations in the function of the serotonergic system during neurodevelopment, whether due to exposure to a drug, the absence of 5-HTT or the manipulation of receptors, lead to behavioural changes in later stages of the individual's life. Therefore, this study assessed whether the increased bioavailability of 5-HT during development, induced by the treatment of pregnant and lactating rats with FLX, would result in neurofunctional alterations (in particular in behaviour and/or the stress response) in the offspring during adolescence and/or adulthood. The stress response was assessed through plasma corticosterone levels and immunohistochemistry for Fos, a protein that is a product of the immediate response gene *c-fos*, expressed in response to neuronal activation and has been used for mapping neural pathways[56].

CHAPTER 2

METHODOLOGY IN ANIMAL MODEL STUDIES

ANIMALS

Virgin female rats were mated (1 male and 3 females per box) throughout the animals' dark period and, on the morning of the following day, pregnancy was diagnosed using a vaginal swab. Rats with the presence of the oestrus phase of the oestrus cycle and the presence of sperm were considered pregnant, and the day of diagnosis was called gestational day 0 (GD0). The pregnant females were then separated and kept in individual boxes in a controlled environment with a temperature of $22\pm2°C$, humidity of $55\pm5\%$, a light/dark cycle of 12h (lights on at 06:00 a.m.) and free access to water and rodent food.

These females were randomly allocated to 2 groups: the control group (CON), which received approximately 0.3mL of water daily by gavage from DG0 onwards; and the treated group (FLX), which received 5mg/Kg/day of FLX (Daforin® oral solution, EMS, Brazil). This dose of FLX was chosen based on preliminary studies carried out in our laboratory which showed that doses higher than 5mg/Kg/day cause maternal toxicity in rats, which is undesirable when a developmental neurotoxicity study is designed. All pregnant rats were weighed to monitor weight gain and adjust the volume of administration.

The day the pups were born was called postnatal day 0 (PND0), and the treatment was continuous and uninterrupted until PND21, when the pups were then weaned and separated into boxes by gender and experimental test, with up to 5 animals per box. At DPN4 the litters were reduced to 10 pups each, keeping an equal number of males and females in the litters when possible. The litters were weighed weekly to monitor weight gain.

The experiments were conducted with pups in adolescence (DPN35) and adulthood (DPN75). All the experimental protocols used in this study were approved by the Ethics Committee for the Use of Animals of the State University of Londrina, Brazil (CEUA 12/11).

In this study we used an acute immobilisation stressor, which consisted of placing the animals in a conical metal tube with openings for ventilation, so that the animal remained restricted inside for 1 hour. The controls (non-stressed animals) remained in their boxes in the vivarium.

After immobilisation stress, the animals intended for plasma corticosterone measurement were guillotined for blood collection in heparinised tubes. Stressed animals (ST groups) and non-stressed animals (NO groups) were guillotined alternately, always between 08:00am and 10:00am, which corresponds approximately to the period when corticosterone levels are lowest (nadir). The aim of choosing this time was to minimise circadian fluctuations in corticosterone levels and increase the sensitivity for detecting possible alterations in the HPA axis induced by maternal exposure to FLX. Adult females had their oestrous phase checked before the experiment using a vaginal swab, and were only subjected to the experiment when they were in oestrus. The blood samples were centrifuged at 3000 rpm for 15 minutes at 4°C and the plasma was separated and frozen at -20°C until corticosterone dosage.

After immobilisation stress, the animals intended for immunohistochemistry were anaesthetised with urethane (1.2g/kg) and then submitted to transcardiac perfusion with saline buffered in 0.2M phosphate buffer (PB) (pH 7.4) followed by 4% paraformaldehyde (PFA) buffered in 0.1M PB (pH 7.4) for fixation. The perfusions of the animals in the ST and NO groups were interspersed and carried out throughout the afternoon (01:00pm to 05:00pm). The brains were removed, post-fixed *overnight* in 4% PFA, and then transferred to vials containing 0.1M PB which remained stored at 4°C until further processing. The brains were placed in a 30% sucrose solution in PB for cryoprotection 48 hours before histological processing.

The brains were cut at 30^m on a freezing microtome (Leica®). The slices were washed in PB and incubated for 16-24h with 1:2000 anti-Fos antibody (*rabbit anti-rat Fos,* Ab-5; Santa Cruz Biotech®) diluted in 0.3% Triton X-100, containing 50^L of normal goat serum. After incubation, the sections were washed 3 times for 10 minutes in PB, and then incubated for 2 hours with 1:200 of biotinylated secondary antibody (*goat anti-rabbit IgG,* Jackson ImmunoResearch®), followed by 3 washes of 10 minutes with PB and then incubated with avidin-biotin complex (1:100; ABC Elite kit, Vector Labs®) for 2 hours. Visualisation was carried out using a mixture of 0.05% diaminobenzidine-0.01% hydrogen peroxide. The sections were then washed in PB and mounted on slides with glycerol-based mounting medium, dried at room temperature, dehydrated with gradual solutions of ethanol followed by xylene, and then covered with permalt (Fisher Scientific®) and a coverslip, for preservation and visualisation under an optical microscope.

Phos-positive neurons were counted bilaterally in two sections of each region analysed: the paraventricular nucleus of the hypothalamus (PVN, bregma - 1.72 to - 1.92 mm) and the amygdala (bregma -1.80 to -2.40 mm). Considering that the amygdala is a heterogeneous collection of nuclei that are activated differently according to the context and type of stress, three subdivisions of the amygdala were analysed separately: the medial amygdala (MeA), the central nucleus of the amygdala (CeA) and the basolateral nucleus of the amygdala (BLA). Each section was photographed at 50x magnification using a photomicroscope coupled to a digital camera, and the photographs were stored on a computer for later digital analysis.

The images were analysed using ImageJ *software* (*National Institutes of Health*, USA). Two sections of each region were analysed bilaterally, generating 4 images of each region for each animal analysed. An average of the number of phospho-positive neurons in each region was calculated, generating a single count for each animal.

Briefly, the region of interest was manually demarcated, within a known area value, and a threshold was set to ensure that only neurone nuclei that could be easily distinguished from the *background were* counted, excluding false positives. A size threshold was also set to eliminate points that were too large or small to be considered neurone nuclei. Once these settings had been adjusted, the *software* counted the number of points in the image (corresponding to the immunolabelled neurons) and this data was then tabulated for later statistical analysis. The result was expressed as the number of immunolabelled neurons/mm^2 of tissue.

Plasma corticosterone levels were measured by radioimmunoassay using the technique described by Elias et al.[57] . Corticosterone was extracted from frozen plasma samples using ethanol (25 µL of plasma + 1mL of ethanol) and then lyophilised. They were then resuspended with 2.5mL of dilution buffer (0.05M Tris-HCl, Sigma®; 0.1M NaCl, Sigma®; 0.1% bovine serum albumin, Sigma®; 0.1% sodium azide, Merck®; pH 8.0). 500 µL of the resuspended samples were taken, in duplicate, to which 100µL of anti-corticosterone antibody (*rabbit anti-rat IgG*, Sigma®) were added, at a dilution of 1:8, and 100µL of tritiated corticosterone ([1,2-3H(N)] - Corticosterone), with an incubation period of 15h.

After incubation, the samples were shaken with 200µL of activated carbon and dextran solution (activated carbon 0.5% - Sigma®; Dextran T70 0.5%, Sigma®) and incubated for 15min at 4°C, then centrifuged at 3000rpm and 4°C for 15min. After centrifugation, 600mL of the supernatant was transferred to scintillation vials containing 5mL of scintillation liquid (ScintiSafe Econo 1 SX20-5, Fischer®) and the radiation (cpm) of the tritiated corticosterone was determined using a liquid scintillation spectrophotometer (Beckman®).

At the same time as the plasma corticosterone concentration was determined, the total concentration of tritiated corticosterone added to each tube (Total) and the non-specific bindings (Blank) were determined. These concentrations were determined following the same procedure described for the samples. For the determination of the non-specific reactions, 600µL of dilution buffer were added in place of the plasma, while for the determination of the total concentration of tritiated corticosterone, 600µL of dilution buffer were added in place of the plasma and, instead of using the activated charcoal suspension, 200μL of dilution buffer were added.

A corticosterone standard curve was made at concentrations of 7.8, 15.6, 31.25, 62.5, 125, 250, 500, 1000 and 2000μL/dL. The curve was subjected to the same procedure for determining the concentration of corticosterone described for the plasma samples, and was plotted using the natural logarithm (ln) of the corticosterone concentration on the x-axis, and on the y-axis the result of the following calculation:

$$\frac{\ln [\text{sample cpm}]}{\ln [\text{cpm of blank-cpm of sample}]}$$

The concentrations of corticosterone present in the samples were calculated by interpolating the readings obtained from the samples (y-axis values) on the standard curve and expressed in μg/dL of plasma corticosterone.

In this test, the animals were separated into individual boxes in which there were two bottles: one containing water and the other containing a 3% sucrose solution, with equal volumes. The sucrose concentration was based on previous studies, which have shown that rodents can perceive sucrose even at concentrations as low as 0.1%, and many studies use sucrose concentrations ranging from 1 to 3% for this test[35] .

The animals had free access to the two bottles for 3 days, and the volume of liquid ingested from each bottle was measured, as well as the animals' weight and, to avoid possible preference for the side of the bottle in the box, the bottles were switched sides daily. The preference for sucrose was then calculated daily as follows:

$$\frac{\text{mL of sucrose solution ingested}}{\text{mL Total Ingested}} \times 100$$

The results were expressed as the total % preference for sucrose, calculated from the sum of each animal's daily preferences.

NOVELTY INDUCED HYPOPHAGIA TEST

This is a test commonly used for mice, and was adapted for rats in this study[58]. The Novelty Induced Hypophagia (NIH) test is based on rodents' innate fear of new and open areas, conflicting with a motivational component (such as hunger or desire for a more palatable food) and has been used to assess behaviours similar to anxiety and depression in rodents.

For this test, the animals were fasted for 24 hours in metabolic cages and then individually placed in the peripheral area of a circular wooden arena (diameter 72cm) which contained 30g of food in its centre. The latency for the animal to start feeding was measured. The tests lasted 5 minutes for the adolescent animals and 15 minutes for the adult animals, due to the fact that the adult animals in both the CON and FLX groups had a longer latency to start feeding. As perinatal treatment with FLX could lead to altered food intake, after the test the animals were returned to the metabolic cage and their food intake was analysed.

their respective cages was also quantified, for the same duration of the test.

The HIN test introduces a paradigm in which there is a conflict between a motivational component of behaviour (hunger) and the rat's fear and anxiety behaviour, which causes it to avoid new and unprotected areas (the central area of an arena). Therefore, the latency to start feeding in the arena reflects the animal's ability to resolve a conflict, which is inversely related to anxiety and depression[58, 59].

STATISTICAL ANALYSIS

The data was initially subjected to an exploratory statistical analysis in which the normal distribution of each variable and the homogeneity of variances were assessed. Parametric analyses (ANOVA, factorial ANOVA or ANOVA for repeated measures) were used for the variables that showed normal distribution and homogeneity of variance. For variables that did not fulfil these two criteria, non-parametric statistical analysis (Kruskal-Wallis) was used. Conclusions were drawn considering a significance level of 95 per cent ($p < 0.05$).

CHAPTER 3

GENERAL TOXICOLOGICAL ASSESSMENT

Treatment with FLX did not alter the weight of the mothers during gestation and lactation (ANOVA for repeated measures, p>0.05) (**Figure 1**), when compared to the CON group. The pups' weight gain was also similar between the two experimental groups (ANOVA for repeated measures, p>0.05) (**Figure 2**). Furthermore, treatment with FLX did not influence the number of pups born alive or dead (data not shown).

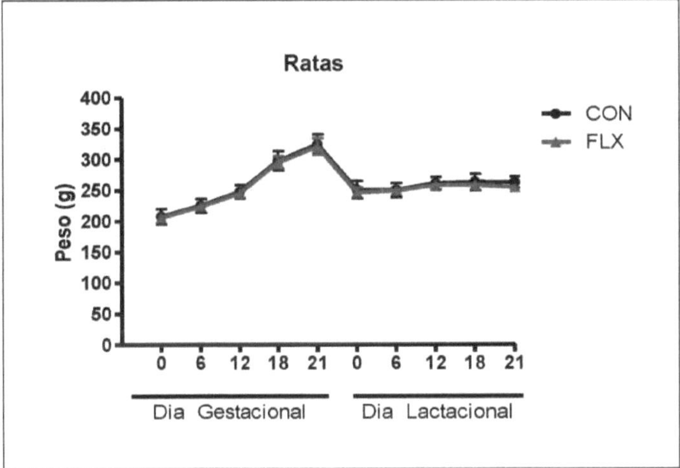

Figura 1. Weight curve of female rats during gestation and lactation. CON, control group (n=40); FLX, fluoxetine group (n=35). Data are means ± EPM. ANOVA for repeated measures, p>0.05.

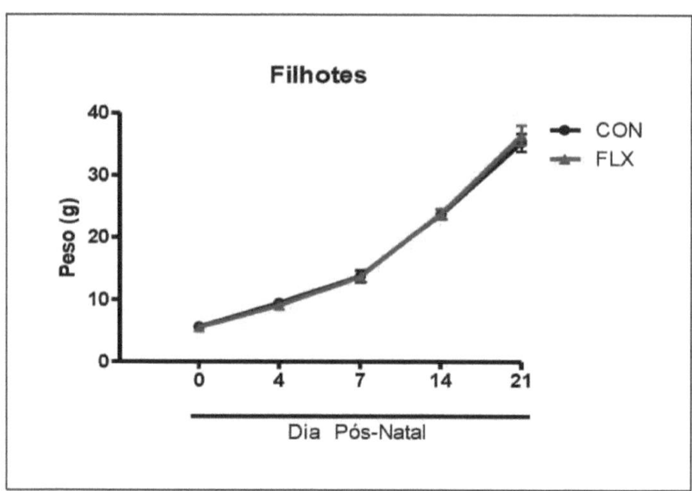

Figura 2. Weight curve of the pups during the lactation period. CON, control group (n=431); FLX, fluoxetine group (n=419). Data are means ± EPM. ANOVA for repeated measures, p>0.05.

IMMUNOHISTOCHEMISTRY FOR PHOS

The count of neurons immunolabelled for Fos was analysed using a non-parametric statistical test, and in this study we used Kruskal-Wallis complemented by Dunn. The data is presented as medians accompanied by minimum and maximum values. The data for males and females, as well as adolescent and adult animals, were all analysed separately since non-parametric analysis does not allow the use of factors.

Males

In adolescent and adult animals (**Figure 3A** and **B**, respectively), the stress protocol significantly increased neuronal activation in the PVN in both the CON and FLX groups. Although this increase did not reach statistical significance in the adolescent CON group and the adult FLX group, it is clear that there is a trend when comparing the respective NO and ST groups (**Figure 4** and **5**). This shows that exposure to FLX during pregnancy and breastfeeding did not alter the stress response of the PVN.

14

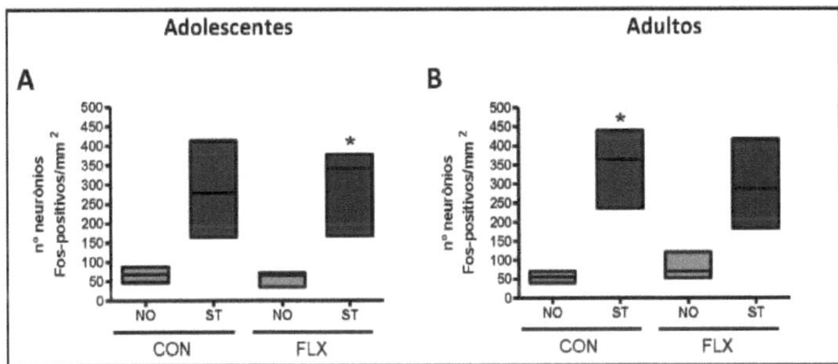

Figura 3. Count of neurons immunolabelled for Fos in the PVN of adolescent and adult male rats in response to the acute stressor of immobilisation. NO, non-stressed group; ST, stressed group; CON, control group; FLX, fluoxetine group. Data are medians ± maximum/minimum of 5-8 animals per group. Kruskal Wallis, *p<0.05 ST compared to respective NO.

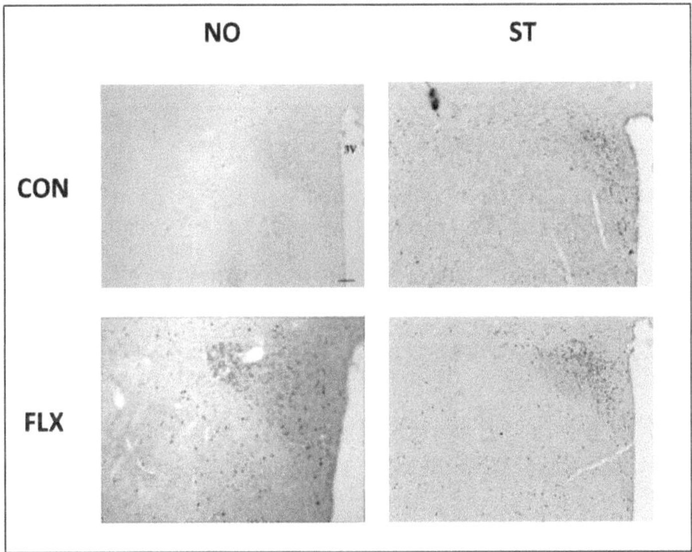

Figura 4. Photomicrographs of the PVN of adolescent male rats. NO, non-stressed group; ST, stressed group; CON, control group; FLX, fluoxetine group. 3V, third ventricle. Scale: 100µm.

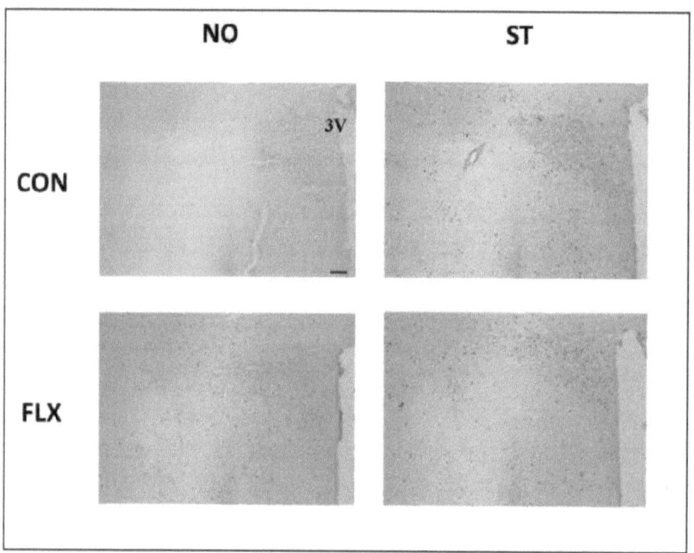

Figure 5 - Photomicrographs of the PVN of adult male rats. NO, non-stressed group; ST, stressed group; CON, control group; FLX, fluoxetine group. 3V, third ventricle. Scale: 100μm.

In the amygdala, we observed different effects according to the nuclei analysed. These differences in amygdala activation in response to a stressor are to be expected, as the amygdala has a complex organisation and responds differently according to the intensity and context of the stressor.

In the BLA of adolescent males, there was stress-induced activation in the CON animals, and we can see that in the group exposed to FLX and subjected to the stressor (FLX ST), there was not only a statistically significant reduction in Fos expression when compared to the group not subjected to the stressor (FLX NO), but there was also a significant difference when compared to the CON group subjected to the stressor (CON ST) (**Figure 6A)**. This shows that exposure to FLX reduced BLA activation against the stressor in adolescent males. In adult males we also observed BLA activation only in the CON group (**Figure 6B)** and, although the FLX ST group was not statistically different from the CON ST group, the data suggest that exposure to FLX may also have reduced BLA responsiveness to the stressor at this age. **Figure 7** and **Figure 8** show photomicrographs of the BLA of adolescent and adult males, respectively.

On the other hand, the CeA (**Figure 6C** and **D)** was unresponsive to the acute stressor of immobilisation (considered a psychological stressor) at both ages, showing that the CeA does not participate in the response to the stress protocol used in this study (**Figure 9** and **10**).

In the MeA, we observed an increase in Fos expression in the CON ST group when compared to the CON NO group in adolescents, although this was not statistically significant (**Figure 6E),** as there was great variability in the data from these groups, which may have hampered the statistical analysis. However, a trend towards increased Fos expression can be observed, and a more detailed analysis of the data indicates that there was a similar induction of activation by the stressor in both groups, with CON ST animals doubling Fos expression compared to CON NO, and FLX ST animals also doubling Fos expression compared to FLX NO, leading to the conclusion that there was indeed stressor-induced activation of the MeA; however, exposure to FLX did not influence this activation. In the adult animals, we observed induction of activation by the stressor in the MeA of the CON animals, but in the FLX animals, we observed a reduction in the stress response of the MeA (**Figure 6F**). We suggest that exposure to FLX decreased the responsiveness of the MeA to the stressor in adult males. Photomicrographs of the MeA can be seen in **Figure 11** and **Figure 12**.

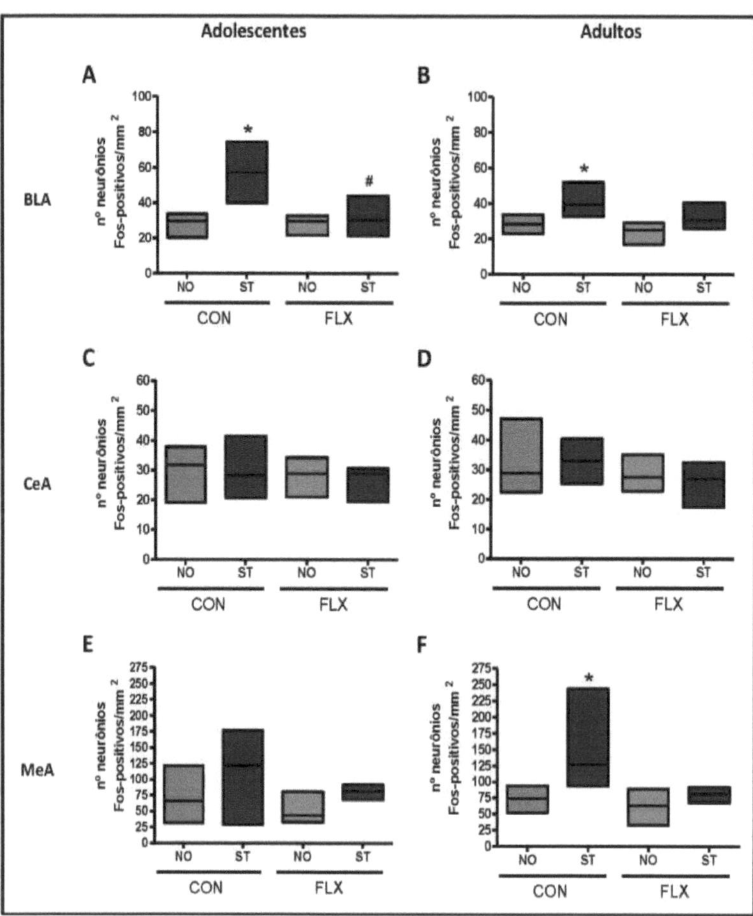

Figura 5. Count of neurons immunolabelled for Fos in different nuclei of the amygdala of adolescent and adult male rats in response to the acute stressor of immobilisation. NO, non-stressed group; ST, stressed group; CON, control group; FLX, fluoxetine group. Data are medians ± maximum/minimum of 5-8 animals per group. Kruskal Wallis, *p<0.05 ST compared to respective NO; #p<0.05 FLX ST compared to CON ST.

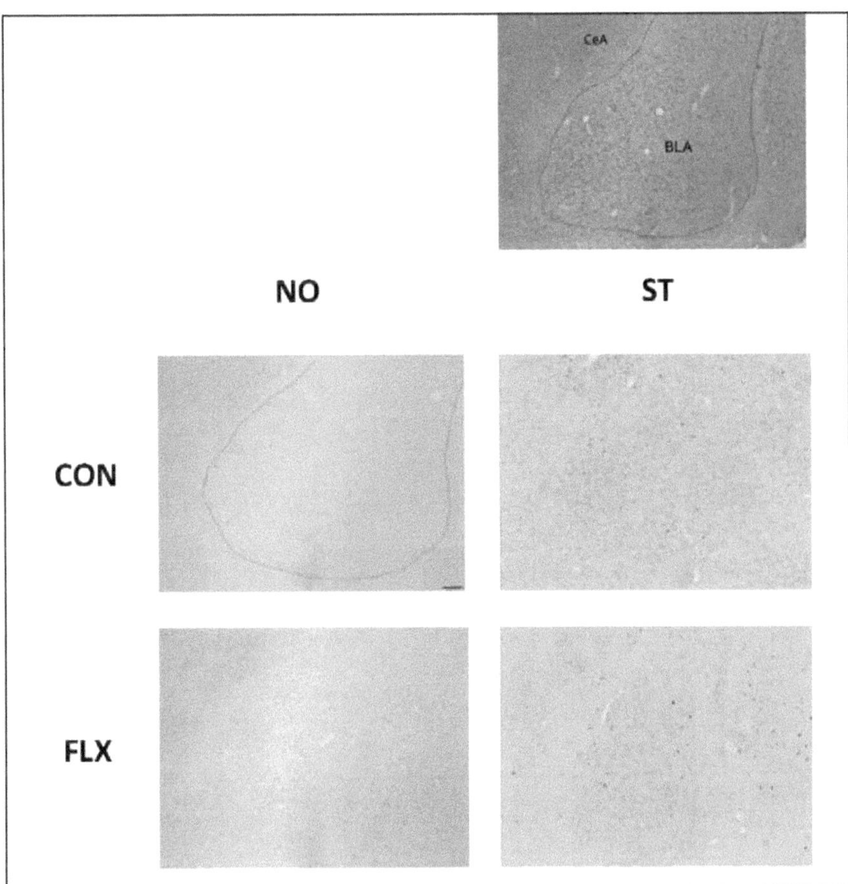

Figure 7. Photomicrographs of the BLA of adolescent male rats. NO, non-stressed group; ST, stressed group; CON, control group; FLX, fluoxetine group. CeA, central nucleus of the amygdala; BLA, basolateral nucleus of the amygdala (demarcated area). Scale: 100μm.

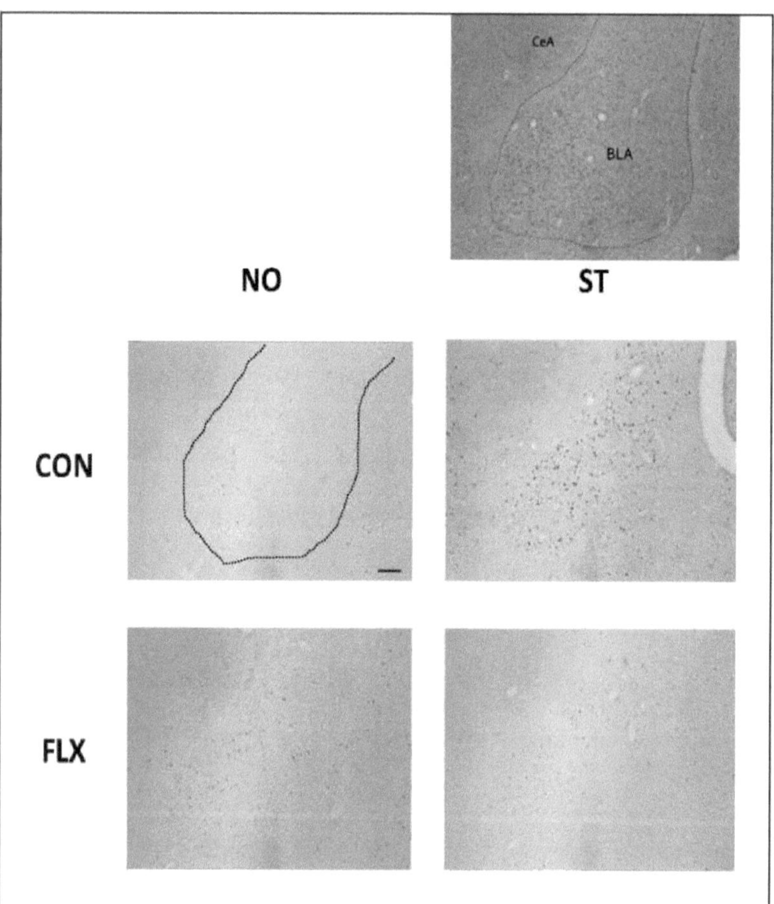

Figure 8. Photomicrographs of the LLA of adult male rats. NO, non-stressed group; ST, stressed group; CON, control group; FLX, fluoxetine group. CeA, central nucleus of the amygdala; BLA, basolateral nucleus of the amygdala (demarcated area). Scale: 100μm.

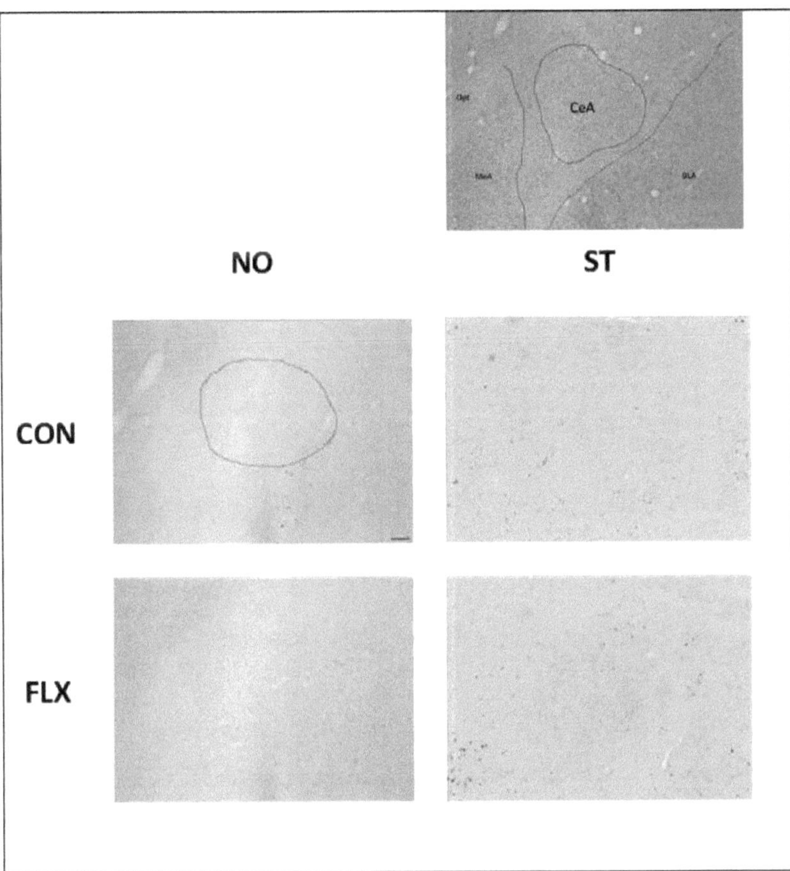

Figure 9. Photomicrographs of the CeA of adolescent male rats. NO, non-stressed group; ST, stressed group; CON, control group; FLX, fluoxetine group. Opt, optic tract; MeA, medial amygdala; BLA, basolateral amygdala; CeA, central amygdala (demarcated area). Scale: 100μm.

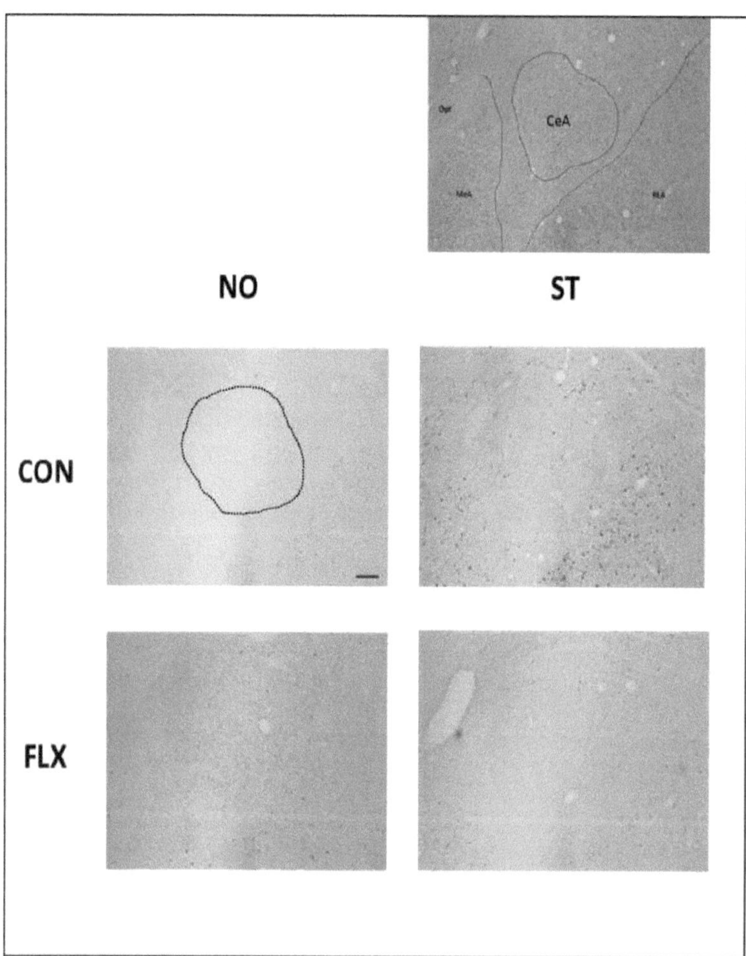

Figure 10. Photomicrographs of the CeA of adult male rats. NO, non-stressed group; ST, stressed group; CON, control group; FLX, fluoxetine group. Opt, optic tract; MeA, medial amygdala; BLA, basolateral amygdala; CeA, central amygdala (demarcated area). Scale: 100µm.

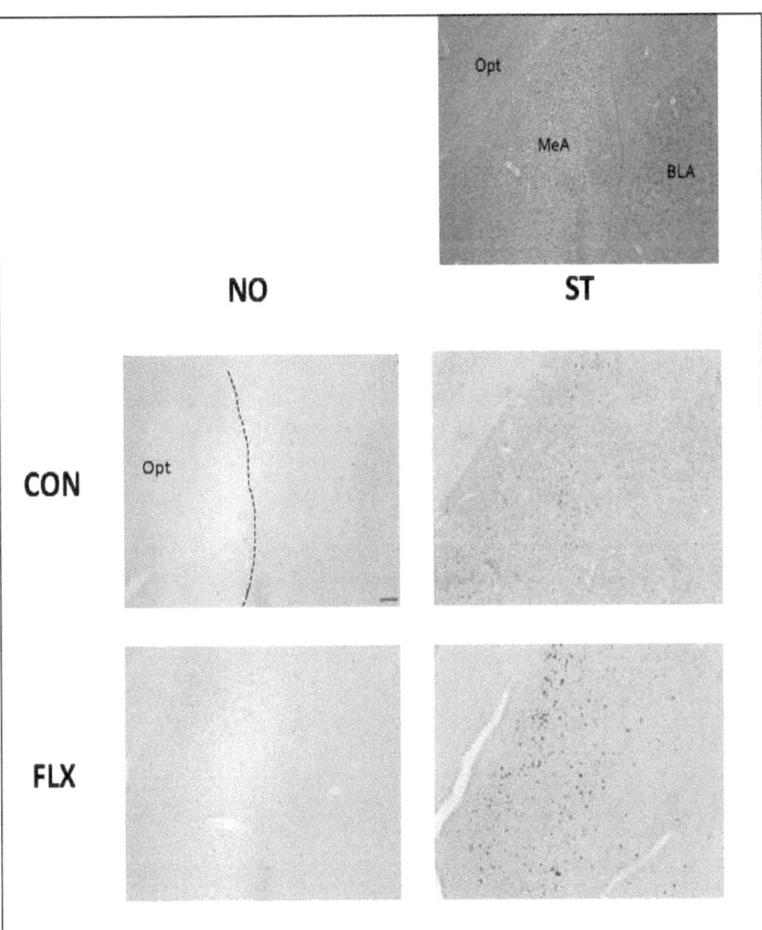

Figure 11. MeA photomicrographs of adolescent male rats. NO, non-stressed group; ST, stressed group; CON, control group; FLX, fluoxetine group. Opt, optic tract; BLA, basolateral nucleus of the amygdala; MeA, medial nucleus of the amygdala (demarcated area). Scale: 100μm.

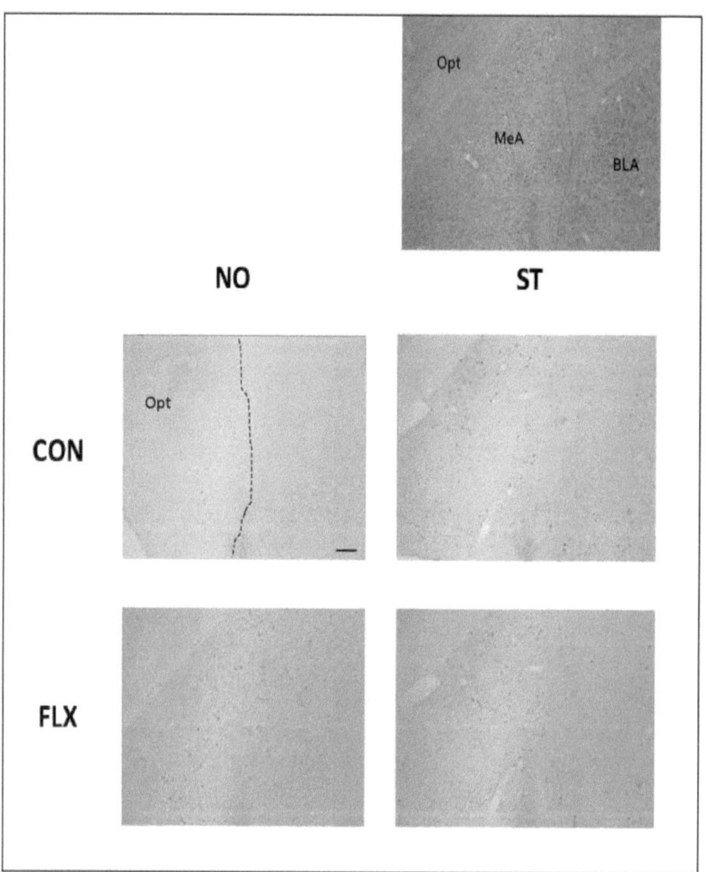

Figure 12. MeA photomicrographs of adult male rats. NO, non-stressed group; ST, stressed group; CON, control group; FLX, fluoxetine group. Opt, optic tract; BLA, basolateral nucleus of the amygdala; MeA, medial nucleus of the amygdala (demarcated area). Scale: 100μm.

Females

Statistical analysis of brain activation in the stress response in CON females showed no statistically significant differences induced by the stressor, when comparing the NO and ST groups, at both ages and in all areas, with the exception of the BLA in adolescents.

In the PVN, although an increase in Fos expression could be observed in the CON ST group when compared to the CON NO group of adolescent and adult rats (**Figure 13**), these increases did not reach statistical significance; on the other hand, in this same nucleus, there was a statistically significant increase in the FLX ST groups when compared to the FLX NO groups, at both ages. We believe that the lack of statistical significance in the CON group was coincidental and suggest that the data should not be interpreted as greater activation in the FLX group (**Figures 14** and **15**).

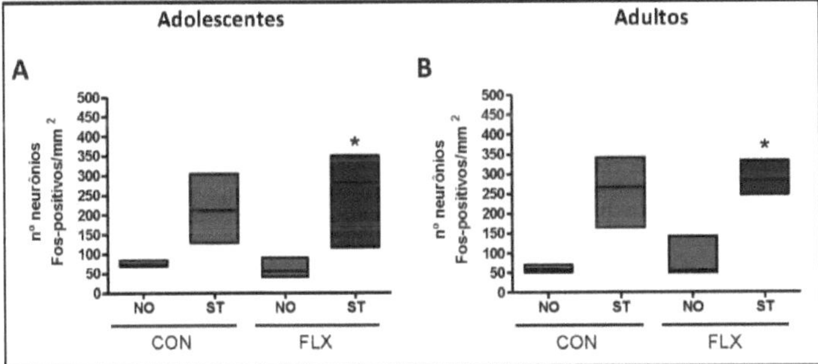

Figure 13. Count of neurons immunolabelled for Fos in the PVN of adolescent and adult female rats in response to the acute stressor of immobilisation. NO, non-stressed group; ST, stressed group; CON, control group; FLX, fluoxetine group. Data are medians ± maximum/minimum of 5-8 animals per group. Kruskal-Wallis, *p<0.05 ST compared to respective NO.

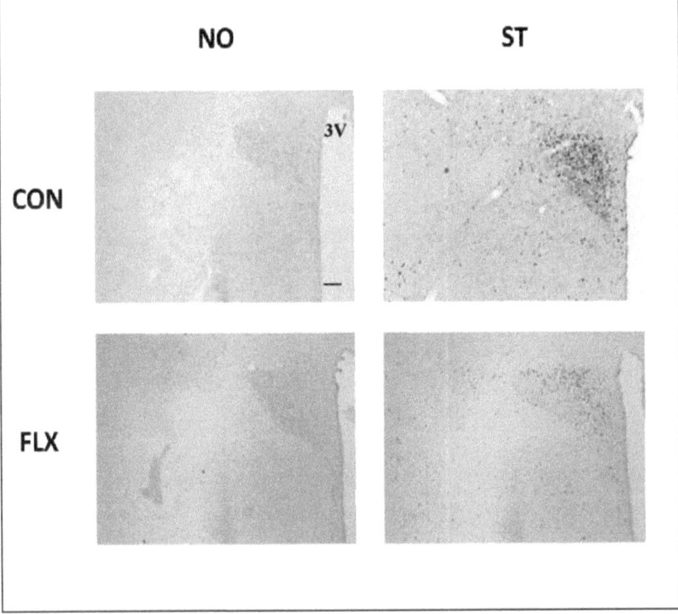

Figure 14. Photomicrographs of the PVN of adolescent female rats. NO, non-stressed group; ST, stressed group; CON, control group; FLX, fluoxetine group. 3V, third ventricle. Scale: 100μm.

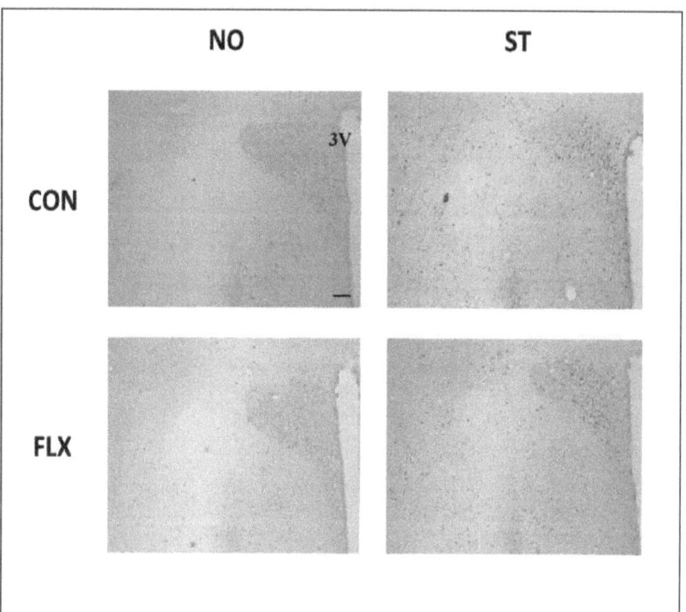

Figure 15. Photomicrographs of the PVN of adult female rats. NO, non-stressed group; ST, stressed group; CON, control group; FLX, fluoxetine group. 3V, third ventricle. Scale: 100μm.

Increased BLA activation was observed in the amygdala of adolescent girls in both the CON and FLX groups (**Figure 16A** and **B**). In adult females, activation of the BLA by the stressor could be observed in the FLX group. Thus, our data show that exposure to FLX during gestation and lactation did not influence the BLA stress response in adolescent or adult rats (**Figure 17** and **18**).

As can be seen in **Figures 16C** and **D**, just like the CeA of males, the CeA of females at both ages was also not activated by the stressor used in this study, again showing that this amygdalar nucleus does not participate in the response to the acute stressor of immobilisation (**Figures 19** and **20**).

In the MeA there was activation by the stressor in all the ST groups, of both ages (**Figure 16E** and **F**), although the increases in the CON groups did not reach statistical significance. Although in the FLX groups the increase was significant, observation of the data suggests that there was no influence of exposure to FLX during gestation and lactation on the MeA activation profile by the stressor (**Figure 21** and **22**). This result contrasts with that observed in adult males, in which there was less

26

responsiveness to the stressor in the MeA of adults exposed to FLX (**Figure 6F**).

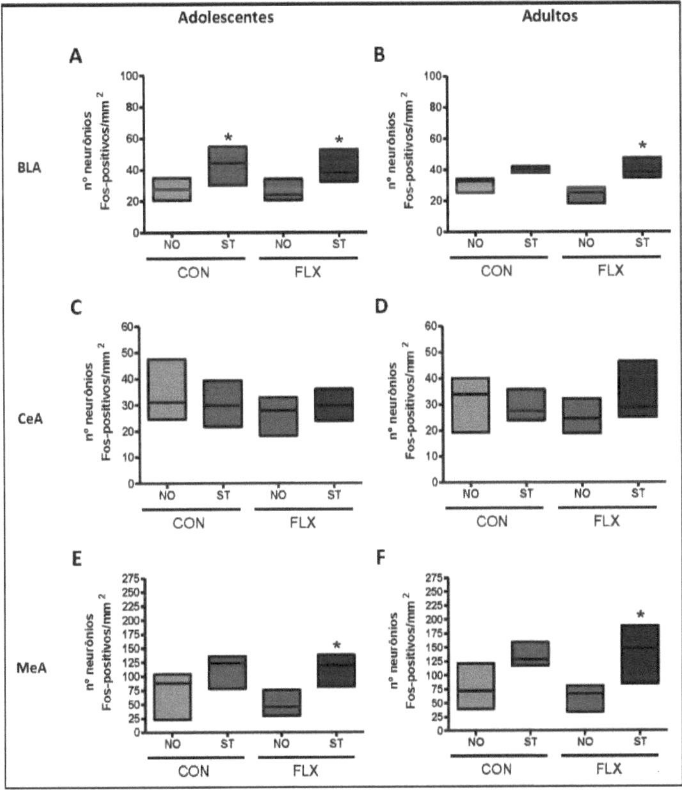

Figure 11. Count of neurons immunolabelled for Fos in different nuclei of the amygdala of adolescent and adult female rats in response to the acute stressor of immobilisation. NO, non-stressed group; ST, stressed group; CON, control group; FLX, fluoxetine group. Data are medians ± maximum/minimum of 5-8 animals per group. Kruskal-Wallis, *p<0.05 ST compared to respective NO.

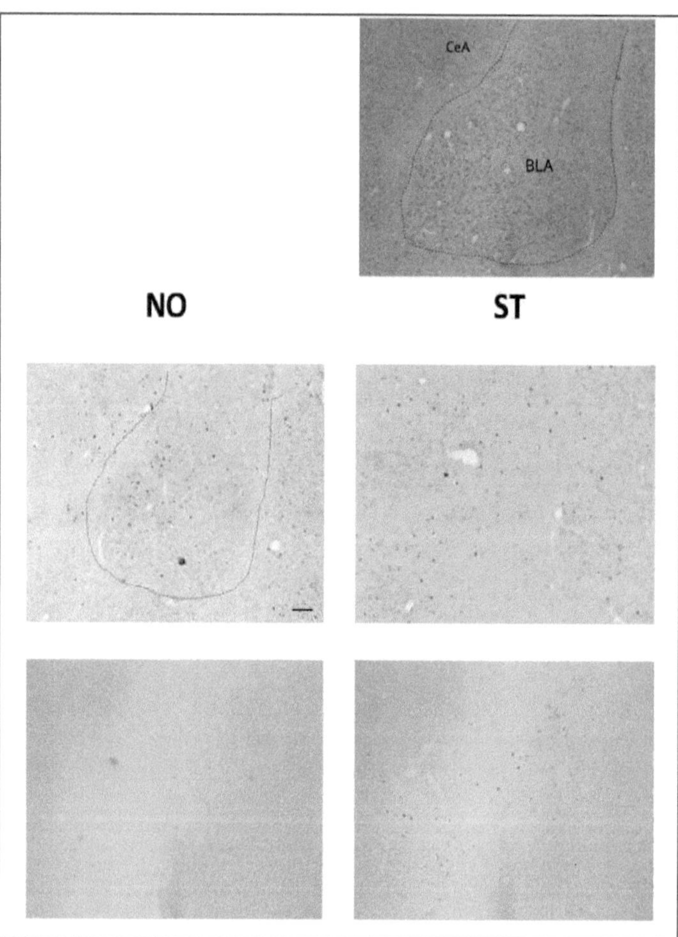

Figure 17. Photomicrographs of the BLA of adolescent female rats. NO, non-stressed group; ST, stressed group; CON, control group; FLX, fluoxetine group. CeA, central nucleus of the amygdala; BLA, basolateral nucleus of the amygdala (demarcated area). Scale: 100μm.

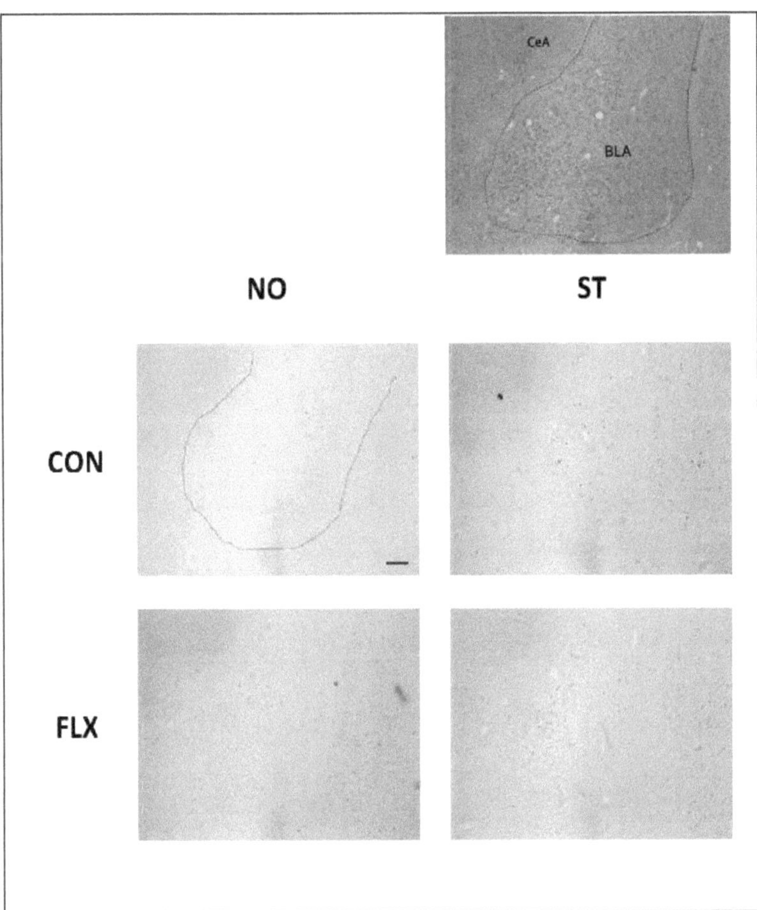

Figure 18. Photomicrographs of the BLA of adult female rats. NO, non-stressed group; ST, stressed group; CON, control group; FLX, fluoxetine group. CeA, central nucleus of the amygdala; BLA, basolateral nucleus of the amygdala (demarcated area). Scale: 100μm.

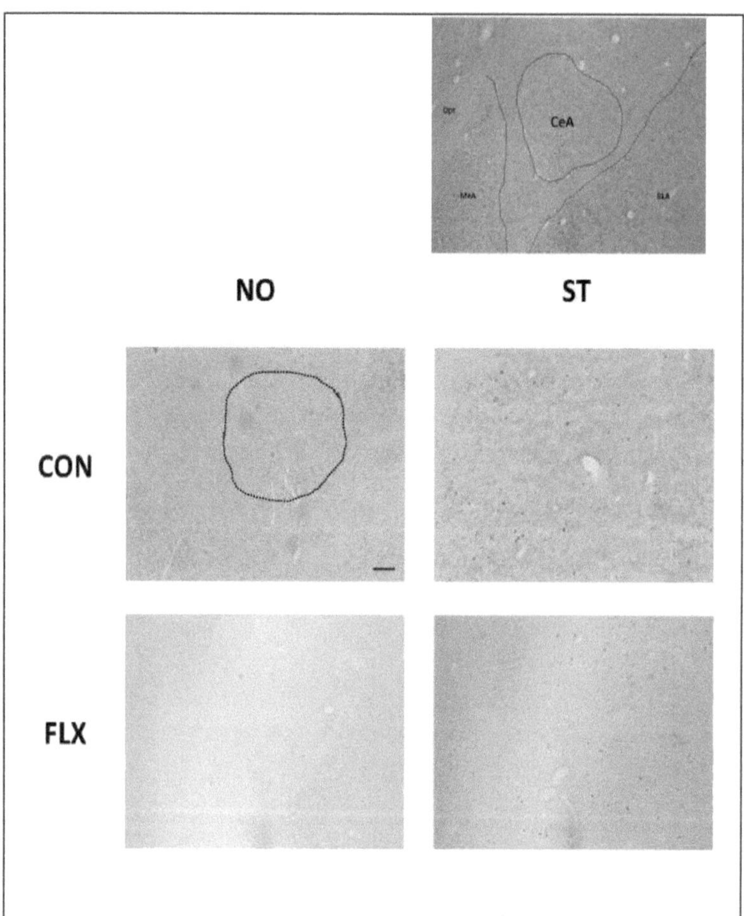

Figure 19. Photomicrographs of the BLA of adolescent female rats. NO, non-stressed group; ST, stressed group; CON, control group; FLX, fluoxetine group. CeA, central nucleus of the amygdala; BLA, basolateral nucleus of the amygdala; Opt, optic tract; MeA, medial amygdala (demarcated area). Scale: 100μm.

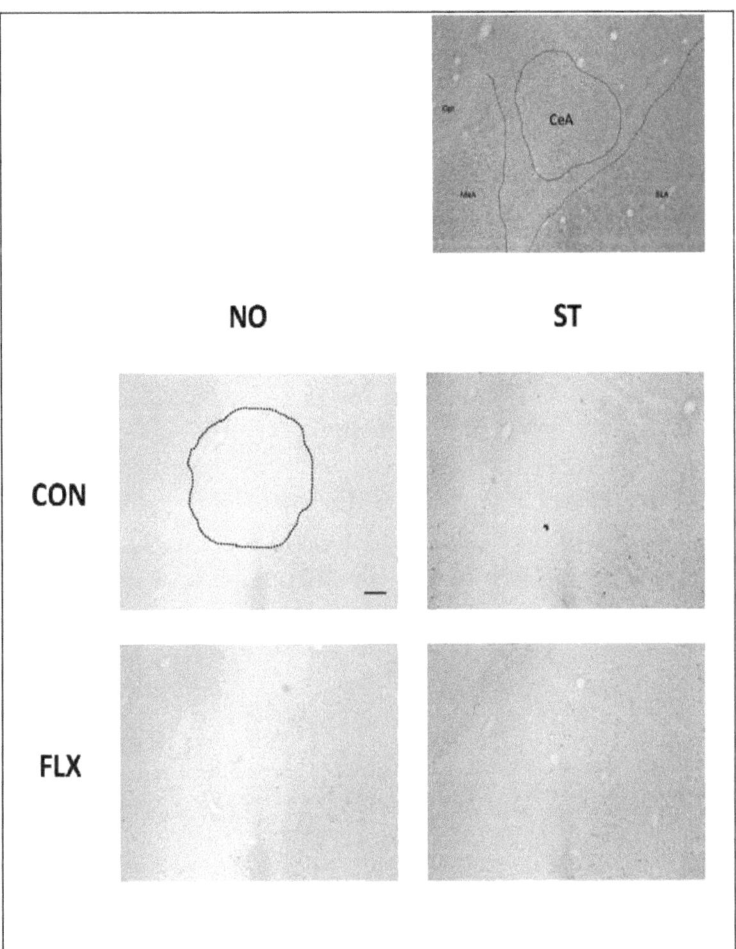

Figure 20. Photomicrographs of the BLA of adolescent female rats. NO, non-stressed group; ST, stressed group; CON, control group; FLX, fluoxetine group. CeA, central nucleus of the amygdala; BLA, basolateral nucleus of the amygdala; Opt, optic tract; MeA, medial amygdala (demarcated area). Scale: 100μm.

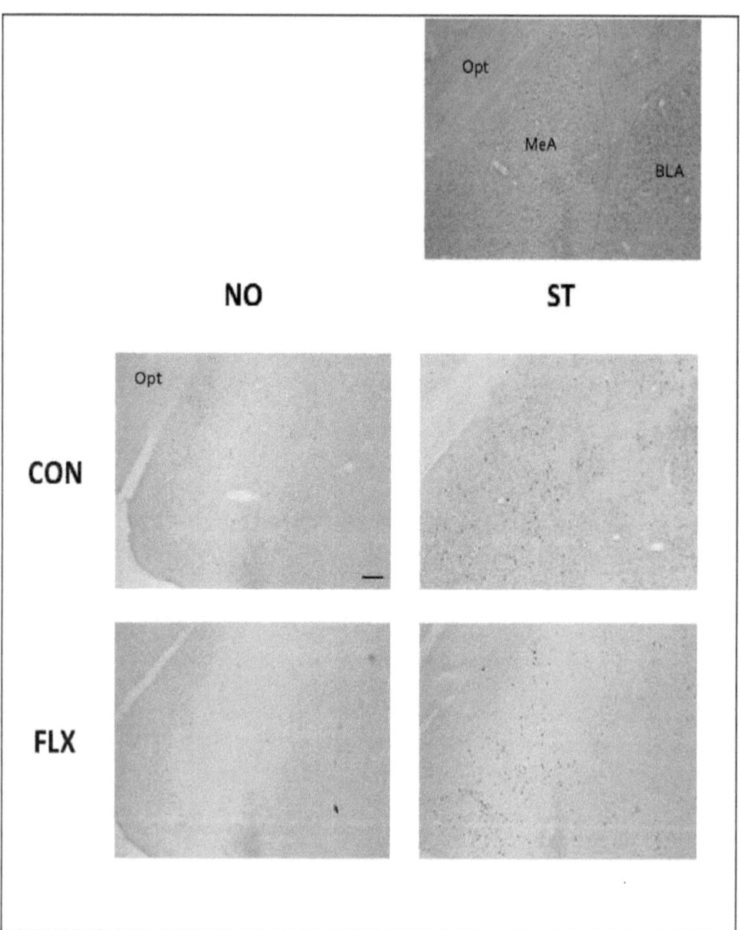

Figure 21. MeA photomicrographs of adolescent female rats. NO, non-stressed group; ST, stressed group; CON, control group; FLX, fluoxetine group. BLA, basolateral nucleus of the amygdala; Opt, optic tract; MeA, medial nucleus of the amygdala (demarcated area). Scale: 100μm.

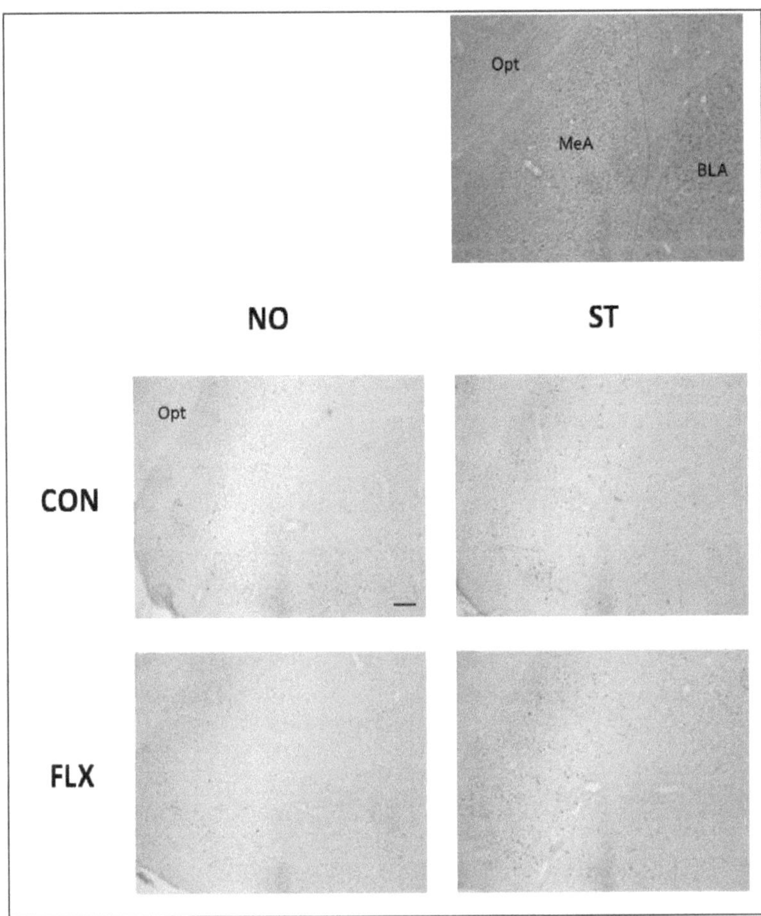

Figure 22. MeA photomicrographs of adult female rats. NO, non-stressed group; ST, stressed group; CON, control group; FLX, fluoxetine group. BLA, basolateral nucleus of the amygdala; Opt, optic tract; MeA, medial nucleus of the amygdala (demarcated area). Scale: 100µm.

PLASMA CORTICOSTERONE

The immobilisation stressor induced a marked increase in plasma corticosterone levels in all the experimental groups (**Figure 23**). A comparison of the ST groups with their respective NO groups showed that the groups were statistically different (Kruskal-Wallis, p<0.05), with the exception of the adolescent females in the control group, in which the greater variability of the NO group's data may have jeopardised the statistical analysis (**Figure 15C**).

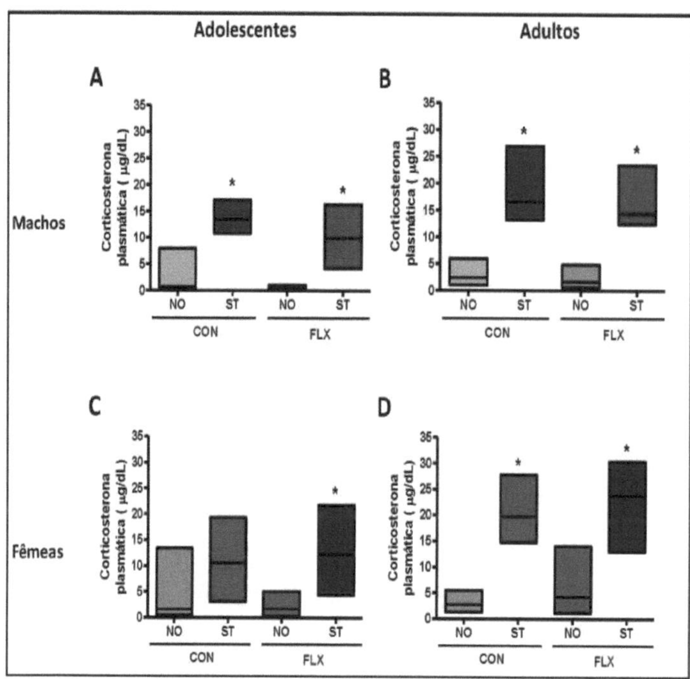

Figura 23. Plasma corticosterone of adolescent and adult male and female rats in response to the acute stressor of immobilisation. NO, non-stressed group; ST, stressed group; CON, control group; FLX, fluoxetine group. Data are medians ± maximum/minimum of 7-12 animals per group. Kruskal-Wallis, *p<0.05 ST compared to respective NO.

Behaviour

The Kruskal-Wallis test showed no significant difference between the groups analysed in the sucrose preference test (**Figure 24**), suggesting that no group showed anhedonia. Total liquid intake was also not significantly different between the groups (data not shown), indicating that exposure to FLX during gestation and breastfeeding does not influence this behaviour or the animals' liquid intake.

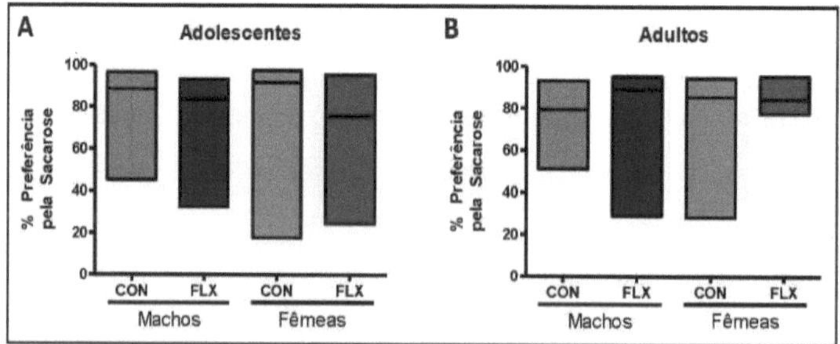

In the HIN test, factorial ANOVA (factors: gender and exposure) showed a significant effect of exposure to FLX on the latency to feed in adolescent animals. Both male and female adolescents exposed to FLX showed lower latency to feed when compared to the CON groups (**Figure 25A**). There was no difference in the feed intake of the animals in their respective metabolic cages (data not shown) suggesting that the effect observed in HIN cannot be attributed to a general reduction in food intake in the animals exposed to FLX. In adult animals, factorial ANOVA did not indicate any significant effect on latency to feed (**Figure 25B**).

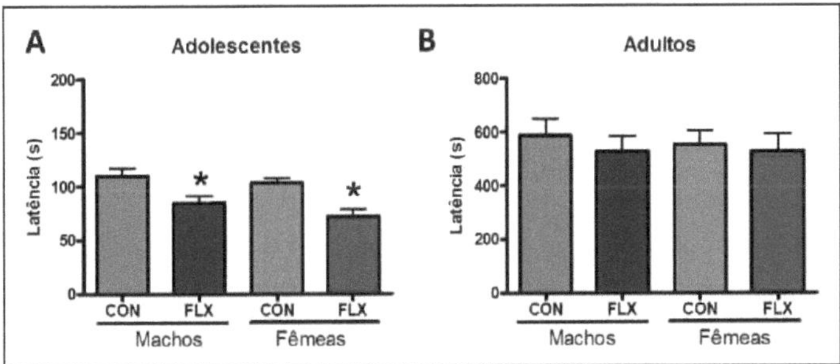

Figure 25. Latency to feed of adolescent and adult male and female rats evaluated in the Novelty-Induced Hypophagia test. Data are means ± SEM of 8-12 animals per group. Factorial ANOVA, * p<0.05 compared to the respective CON group.

CHAPTER 4

The lack of effect of FLX on maternal weight, number of pups born alive and dead and pup weight at birth and during lactation shows that the FLX exposure regime used in this study did not induce general toxicity, which is desirable in studies evaluating functional effects after exposure to drugs during the development of the organism.

Analysing the immunohistochemistry data together, we see that there is a gender difference in the stress response. The data from the CON groups indicate that females have less neuronal activation than males in response to the acute stressor of immobilisation. Gender differences in the stress response were also described by Mitsushima et al.[60] . These authors reported that females have less basal 5-HT in the BLA when compared to males, which could be related to the greater emotional vulnerability of females. However, when exposed to an acute restraint stressor, females show higher levels of 5-HT and dopamine in the amygdala, suggesting that females have differences in the neural connections of the stress system and are naturally better able to resolve a stressful situation than males. In addition, differences in basal 5-HT and dopamine levels in the brains of males and females have also been demonstrated[61]
.

The effect of exposure to FLX on Fos expression was also shown to be gender-dependent. In general terms, males in the FLX groups showed less activation of the amygdala by the stressor, while females in the FLX groups showed increased responsiveness to the stressor in the same area. It is interesting to mention that, in addition to differences in the serotonergic system of males and females, as mentioned in the previous paragraph, we found studies in the literature that report distinct functional differences between genders in animals exposed perinatally to FLX. In studies evaluating both genders exposed to FLX (mice, 7.5mg/Kg/day, gavage, DG0 - DPN21), only the females showed depressive behaviour (LISBOA et al., 2007) and a reduction in behavioural responses mediated by the dopaminergic system[22]. Perinatal exposure to other classes of drugs that do not act directly on the serotonergic system also leads to gender-specific differences. Frieder and Grimm[62] showed that perinatal administration of diazepam (rats, 10mg/Kg/day, subcutaneous, DG8-14 or DG14-20) alters brain levels of 5-HT differently in males and females. Taken together, these facts show not only a naturally distinct serotonergic system, but also that it responds differently not only to manipulations of the serotonergic system, but also to manipulations of other systems.

The amygdala projects to the medial prefrontal cortex and receives other projections from it that modulate its activity. This circuit is responsible for establishing a flexible stress response, according to the context of the stressor, leading to a *bottom-up response,* characterised by the amygdala's control over the cortex, or a *top-down* response, in which the cortex exerts inhibitory control over the amygdala[50, 63, 64]. Both types of responses are necessary for the individual to adapt to the context of the stressor, leading to an optimised response for each situation and allowing for better chances of survival. Males seem to show a predominance of *top-down response*, while females show a predominance of *bottom-up* stress response, although these differences in the regulation of stress circuitry seem to culminate in similar psychophysiological effects, as hypothesised in animal and human studies[49, 65]. Based on our data, we suggest that exposure to FLX may have impaired the formation of neural connections between the amygdala and the prefrontal cortex, altering the differential regulation of the stress response between genders, since we observed in this study that males exposed to FLX during gestation and breastfeeding showed a decrease in responsiveness to the stressor, in general terms, while females had an increase in this responsiveness, when compared to CON animals.

The MeA is an output nucleus of the stress response in the amygdala, projecting to other areas such as the BNST and hypothalamus, and responds mainly to psychological stressors; it undergoes plasticity through the experience of stressful events during life, and is classified as a non-cortical nucleus, as is the CeA, whereas the BLA is classified as a cortical nucleus[66]. It can be seen that exposure to FLX altered the intra-amygdalar stress response circuit in males, as adolescent males showed reduced BLA activation but normal MeA activation, while adult males showed exactly the opposite effects, i.e. normal BLA activation and reduced MeA activation. This suggests that exposure to FLX led to alterations in the stress neural circuitry in an age-dependent manner.

Interestingly, adolescent male rats exposed to FLX (10mg/Kg/day, subcutaneous, DG2-DG21) show increased expression of 5-HTT in the BLA and MeA, an effect that does not appear in adult males[67]. Furthermore, both acute and chronic stress induce the formation of dendritic spines in the BLA[66] causing permanent changes in the intra-amygdalar circuitry, a process that is also modulated by 5-HT[18, 68]. Therefore, if exposure to FLX led to reduced levels of 5-HT in the BLA and MeA by increasing the expression of 5-HTT during adolescence, interference is expected in the plasticity processes of the BLA and MeA, which depend on the formation of dendritic spines in cortical neurons, which could impair the formation of memories related to stressful events. Thus, a decrease in BLA activity during adolescence could impair memory formation to stressful events, which in turn would lead to a decrease in the MeA response in adulthood.

With regard to CeA, in this study we observed that it did not respond to the stressor used. There is evidence that the brain is able to recognise two main classes of stressors: physical stressors, which are those that cause a direct threat to life (such as bleeding or infection), and psychological stressors, which are those that cause worry and anxiety but do not immediately threaten the individual's life (such as tests and embarrassing social situations)[47]. Although there is debate about how to model these two types of stressors in animals, or even whether there is such a differentiation in the brain, data from the literature has shown that different stressor protocols do lead to different activations of the stress neural circuitry. The results of our study corroborate reports that the amygdala is capable of differentiating between psychological and physical stressors, with the CeA being responsive only to physical stressors[69].

The PVN is also an important nucleus involved in the stress response. It exerts control over the HPA axis and, because it is one of the main controllers of the axis, it receives many projections from various brain areas, including the amygdala, BNST and prefrontal cortex, which usually interact with inhibitory interneurons close to the PVN[70] . Regions of the limbic system and the amygdala, when activated, lead to disinhibition of the PVN, thus allowing the HPA axis to act in the face of a stressor. On the other hand, brainstem nuclei, such as the raphe nuclei and ventral tegmental area, connect directly to the PVN via glutamatergic neurons and activate it directly in response to a stressful event[70] . In this study, we observed a marked increase in the activation of this nucleus in all the experimental groups in the face of the stressor, proving the efficacy of the protocol used, as well as the lack of effect of exposure to FLX on the activation of the PVN. It is possible that 5-HT modifies some projections to the PVN during development, but as the PVN is a nucleus that integrates various responses not only to stress but also to endocrine and other behaviours, such as food intake, subtle changes in its functioning may not result in apparent functional effects. However, these possible alterations to the PVN could increase susceptibility to the development of endocrine or neuropsychiatric pathologies. In fact, abnormalities in growth and weight gain have been reported in studies of animals and humans exposed to SSRIs during pregnancy and lactation[71] .

We demonstrated the efficiency of our stressor protocol both by activating the PVN and by the marked increase in plasma corticosterone levels in the stressed rats. However, we observed no effect of exposure to FLX during gestation and lactation on the increase in plasma corticosterone in response to the stressor. 5-HT is closely related not only to the development of the HPA axis, but also to its functioning[72] , and several evidences of alterations in the HPA axis by manipulation of the serotonergic system are found in the literature. Clinical research has shown a reduction in basal salivary cortisol levels in neonates exposed to SSRIs[73] , as well as attenuation of the acute stress response[74, 75] . In sheep, exposure to FLX at a dose of 98.5 iig/Kg/day intravenously during gestation results in increased plasma cortisol levels and other changes in the behaviour of foetuses[76] , and rats exposed to FLX (5mg/Kg/day, DPN1-21, via osmotic minipumps) have reduced plasma corticosterone levels in response to stress .[77]

In an elegant study, Pawluski et al.[78] demonstrated a reduction in plasma corticosterone levels in adolescent rats (DPN 39-42) exposed to FLX during the lactational period (5mg/Kg/day, via osmotic mini-pumps in lactating females), as well as a reduction in the expression of glucocorticoid receptors in the hippocampus of these animals. These effects were not observed in the female pups, corroborating our results which show a marked gender difference in the effects of perinatal exposure to FLX. These authors suggest that the difference in relation to the HPA axis may be due to circulating sex hormones, as other studies have shown modulation of the HPA axis by oestradiol[79] , but point out that this difference may be neural, since males and females have different levels of 5-HT in various brain regions[61] . As we did not observe any effect of exposure to FLX on the intensity of activation of the PVN by the immobilisation stressor, the fact that we did not find changes in circulating corticosterone levels would be expected. However, it is important to note that in this study, the route of administration and period of exposure used were different to the protocol used by Pawluski et al, which may explain the discrepancy in results between the two studies. It is also important to mention that, during the exploratory analysis of the data, we observed an apparent reduction in plasma corticosterone levels in response to the stressor in adolescent males exposed to FLX, but statistical analysis of the data showed no significant difference. It is possible that by increasing the sampling of the groups to try to reduce the variability of the data, we could find significant differences.

In relation to the behaviours analysed in this study, exposure to FLX did not influence the animals' ability to feel pleasure, but it did reduce anxiety/depressive-like behaviour in adolescent males and females. Anhedonia is a symptom of depression, characterised by the inability to feel pleasure, and has been mimicked in some animal models, such as the sucrose preference test, which has construct validity (i.e. animals exposed to factors that lead to depression show anhedonia in this test) and face validity (i.e. it is able to mimic a symptom observed in people with depression). The absence of anhedonia observed in this study as a result of exposure to FLX is in line with studies in the literature carried out with 5-HTT knockout mice[35, 80] , which also develop in the presence of increased levels of 5-HT. It is known that animals exposed perinatally to

FLX show disturbances in the reward system[81] , but it is not clear whether this alteration results in increased or decreased circuit activity.

In the HIN test we have a complex behavioural situation in which it is assumed that the animal will be motivated by hunger to approach the food, but the location of the food in an unprotected place in an unknown arena induces conflict in the animal, and consequently anxiety. In fact, the anti-conflict potential of various drugs has been shown to be positively correlated with their clinical efficacy as anxiolytics[82] . Furthermore, as the ability to resolve conflicts is implicated in the etiology of depression (a greater ability to resolve conflicts reflects a better resolution of stressful situations), the HIN test has also been used to evaluate antidepressant drugs. Therefore, by measuring the latency to eat, similar anxiety and depressive behaviours can be assessed. The reduction in latency in this test therefore suggests that these animals show a reduction in similar anxiety/depression behaviours when they are adolescents. Similar effects have been described in adult female mice (DPN 73-83) assessed in the elevated cross maze and forced swim tests, after exposure to FLX (25mg/Kg/day, drinking water, DG15- DPN12)[83] and another author reports that there is no effect of exposure to FLX during pregnancy on the behaviour of adult male and female mice, assessed in various behavioural tests, using an exposure regime with doses ranging from 1- 12mg/Kg/day, gavage, DG7-DG20[4, 83] . However, increased behaviours similar to anxiety and depression have also been reported after exposure to high levels of 5-HT during development in rodents .[18, 21, 25, 27, 32]

The apparent inconsistency of the effects reported in studies assessing anxiety and depression in animals exposed perinatally to FLX or other SSRIs may be due to differences in exposure protocols, such as the use of different doses, route of administration, treatment period, gender, animal species used or behavioural tests carried out. However, we must also consider that both anxiety and depression are neuropsychiatric diseases that involve a myriad of symptoms[84] and the parameters assessed in animal models reflect only some of them. Therefore, it is difficult to draw conclusions about the effects of perinatal exposure to increased levels of 5-HT in relation to these behaviours.

Finally, in relation to the HIN test, it is worth noting that the animals' response in this test may also be related to impulsiveness. The time it takes the animal to approach the food could be driven not by a greater ability to resolve the conflict, but by the animal's greater impulsiveness, i.e. a greater predisposition to take risks. Following this reasoning, in the HIN test, if the animal is more impulsive, it will have a shorter latency to feed. Supporting this idea, in our study we observed a time 5 to 6 times longer in adult animals compared to adolescent animals, which are known to be more impulsive[85] . Therefore, at the moment, we cannot say whether the results observed in the adolescent animals in the FLX group (i.e. reduced latency to feed) reflect an increase in impulsivity or a reduction in similar anxiety/depression behaviours.

CHAPTER 5

The impact of perinatal exposure to SSRIs has been a growing concern since the introduction of SSRIs to the market in the late 1980s, when reports of neonatal abstinence syndrome in neonates of mothers being treated with these drugs began to appear. Experiments conducted on rodents and sheep to assess the effect of perinatal exposure to SSRIs have revealed neurofunctional changes in the foetus and offspring; but there is controversy between these studies, as not all have reported the same neurofunctional effects and sometimes have shown discrepant and paradoxical effects, leaving it open as to whether the effects are transient or whether permanent changes occur in the developing brain, leading to altered function in adulthood.

In this study, it was observed that the exposure of rats to FLX during neurodevelopment caused alterations in behaviour, as well as an altered stress response during adolescence. However, these effects appear to be transient, as they did not manifest in adulthood. It was also shown that, compared to males, females exhibit important differences in the stress response, indicating a difference in the neural connections involved in the stress response between males and females. Additionally, the outcomes of perinatal exposure to FLX represent an interconnection between psychological, genetic, pharmacological and environmental factors, making it difficult to establish a "main effect" of this exposure, and the clinical implications and importance of these effects will have to be determined in the future. It is important to emphasise that extrapolating the results to define the safety of FLX in relation to developmental neurotoxicity for humans is a complex task, as many factors can interfere in experimental studies, which interact in a complex way to determine the functioning of the individual's organism in the adult phase.

There is still a lot of work to be done to fully understand the role of perinatal exposure to SSRIs in the context of development, and the impacts that this exposure, added to maternal mood swings, could have later on in the individual's life.

BIBLIOGRAPHICAL REFERENCES

1. Kessler, R.C., et al, *Lifetime prevalence and age-of-onset distributions of DSM-IV disorders in the National Comorbidity Survey Replication.* Arch Gen Psychiatry, 2005. **62**(6): p. 593-602.

2. Austin, M.P., S. Kildea, and E. Sullivan, *Maternal mortality and psychiatric morbidity in the perinatal period: challenges and opportunities for prevention in the Australian setting.* Med J Aust, 2007. **186**(7): p. 364-7.

3. Gentile, S., *Neurodevelopmental effects of prenatal exposure to psychotropic medications.* Depress Anxiety, 2011. **27**(7): p. 675-86.

4. Vorhees, C.V., et al, *A developmental neurotoxicity evaluation of the effects of prenatal exposure to fluoxetine in rats.* Fundam Appl Toxicol, 1994. **23**(2): p. 194-205.

5. Lattimore, K.A., et al, *Selective serotonin reuptake inhibitor (SSRI) use during pregnancy and effects on the fetus and newborn: a meta-analysis.* J Perinatol, 2005. **25**(9): p. 595-604.

6. Wong, D.T., et al, *A selective inhibitor of serotonin uptake: Lilly 110140, 3-(p-trifluoromethylphenoxy)-N-methyl-3-phenylpropylamine.* Life Sci, 1974. **15**(3): p. 471-9.

7. Nonacs, R. and L.S. Cohen, *Assessment and treatment of depression during pregnancy: an update.* Psychiatr Clin North Am, 2003. **26**(3): p. 547-62.

8. Hendrick, V., et al, *Placental passage of antidepressant medications.* Am J Psychiatry, 2003. **160**(5): p. 993-6.

9. Pohland, R.C., et al., *Placental transfer and foetal distribution of fluoxetine in the rat.* Toxicol Appl Pharmacol, 1989. **98**(2): p. 198-205.

10. Hendrick, V., et al, *Fluoxetine and norfluoxetine concentrations in nursing infants and breast milk.* Biol Psychiatry, 2001. **50**(10): p. 775-82.

11. Suri, R., et al, *Estimates of nursing infant daily dose of fluoxetine through breast milk.* Biol Psychiatry, 2002. **52**(5): p. 446-51.

12. Heikkinen, T., et al, *Pharmacokinetics of fluoxetine and norfluoxetine in pregnancy and lactation.* Clin Pharmacol Ther, 2003. **73**(4): p. 330-7.

13. Iqbal, M., et al, *Placental drug transporters and their role in foetal protection.* Placenta, 2012. **33**(3): p. 137-42.

14. Zhong, P., E.Y. Yuen, and Z. Yan, *Modulation of neuronal excitability by serotonin-NMDA interactions in prefrontal cortex.* Mol Cell Neurosci, 2008. **38**(2): p. 290-9.

15. Yuen, E.Y., et al, *Serotonin 5-HT1A receptors regulate NMDA receptor channels through a microtubule-dependent mechanism.* J Neurosci, 2005. **25**(23): p. 5488-501.

16. Lauder, J.M., *Ontogeny of the serotonergic system in the rat: serotonin as a developmental signal.* Ann N Y Acad Sci, 1990. **600**: p. 297-313; discussion 314.

17. Whitaker-Azmitia, P.M., et al, *Serotonin as a developmental signal.* Behav Brain Res, 1996. **73**(1-2): p. 19-29.

18. Homberg, J.R., D. Schubert, and P. Gaspar, *New perspectives on the neurodevelopmental effects of SSRIs.* Trends Pharmacol Sci, 2010. **31**(2): p. 605.

19. Kiyasova, V. and P. Gaspar, *Development of raphe serotonin neurons from specification to guidance.* Eur J Neurosci, 2011. **34**(10): p. 1553-62.

20. Bonnin, A. and P. Levitt, *Fetal, maternal, and placental sources of serotonin and new implications for developmental programming of the brain.* Neuroscience, 2011. **197**: p. 1-7.

21. Popa, D., et al, *Lasting syndrome of depression produced by reduction in serotonin uptake during postnatal development: evidence from sleep, stress, and behaviour.* J Neurosci, 2008. **28**(14): p. 3546-54.

22. Favaro, P.N., L.C. Costa, and E.G. Moreira, *Maternal fluoxetine treatment decreases behavioural response to dopaminergic drugs in female pups.* Neurotoxicol Teratol, 2008. **30**(6): p. 487-94.

23. Gerardin, D.C., et al, *Sexual behaviour, neuroendocrine, and neurochemical aspects in male rats exposed prenatally to stress.* Physiol Behav, 2005. **84**(1): p. 97-104.

24. Gouvea, T.S., et al., *Maternal exposure to the antidepressant fluoxetine impairs sexual motivation in adult male mice.* Pharmacol Biochem Behav, 2008. **90**(3): p. 416-9.

25. Ansorge, M.S., et al, *Early-life blockade of the 5-HT transporter alters emotional behaviour in adult mice.* Science, 2004. **306**(5697): p. 879-81.

26. Hansen, H.H., C. Sanchez, and E. Meier, *Neonatal administration of the selective serotonin reuptake inhibitor Lu 10-134-C increases forced swimming-induced immobility in adult rats: a putative animal model of depression?* J Pharmacol Exp Ther, 1997. **283**(3): p. 1333-41.

27. Lisboa, S.F., et al., *Behavioral evaluation of male and female mice pups exposed to fluoxetine during pregnancy and lactation.* Pharmacology, 2007. **80**(1): p. 4956.

28. Alexandre, C., et al, *Early life blockade of 5-hydroxytryptamine 1A receptors normalizes sleep and depression-like behaviour in adult knock-out mice lacking the serotonin transporter.* J Neurosci, 2006. **26**(20): p. 5554-64.

29. Kalueff, A.V., et al, *Hypolocomotion, anxiety and serotonin syndrome-like behaviour contribute to the complex phenotype of serotonin transporter knockout mice.* Genes Brain Behav, 2007. **6**(4): p. 389-400.

30. Holmes, A. and A.R. Hariri, *The serotonin transporter gene-linked polymorphism and negative emotionality: placing single gene effects in the context of genetic background and environment.* Genes Brain Behav, 2003. **2**(6): p. 332-5.

31. Olivier, J.D., et al, *A study in male and female 5-HT transporter knockout rats: an animal model for anxiety and depression disorders.* Neuroscience, 2008.

152(3): p. 573-84.

32. Olivier, J.D., et al., *Fluoxetine administration to pregnant rats increases anxiety-related behaviour in the offspring.* Psychopharmacology (Berl), 2011. **217**(3): p. 419-32.

33. Ansorge, M.S., E. Morelli, and J.A. Gingrich, *Inhibition of serotonin but not norepinephrine transport during development produces delayed, persistent perturbations of emotional behaviours in mice.* J Neurosci, 2008. **28**(1): p. 199207.

34. Mosienko, V., et al, *Exaggerated aggression and decreased anxiety in mice deficient in brain serotonin.* Transl Psychiatry, 2012. **2**: p. e122.

35. Kalueff, A.V., P.S. Gallagher, and D.L. Murphy, *Are serotonin transporter knockout mice 'depressed'?: hypoactivity but no anhedonia.* Neuroreport, 2006. **17**(12): p. 1347-51.

36. Uher, R., *The implications of gene-environment interactions in depression: will cause inform cure?* Mol Psychiatry, 2008. **13**(12): p. 1070-8.

37. Homberg, J.R., et al, *Adaptations in pre- and postsynaptic 5-HT1A receptor function and cocaine supersensitivity in serotonin transporter knockout rats.* Psychopharmacology (Berl), 2008. **200**(3): p. 367-80.

38. Homberg, J.R., et al., *Acute and constitutive increases in central serotonin levels reduce social play behaviour in peri-adolescent rats.* Psychopharmacology (Berl), 2007. **195**(2): p. 175-82.

39. Holmes, A., D.L. Murphy, and J.N. Crawley, *Reduced aggression in mice lacking the serotonin transporter.* Psychopharmacology (Berl), 2002. **161**(2): p. 160-7.

40. Olivier, J.D., et al, *Serotonin transporter deficiency in rats contributes to impaired object memory.* Genes Brain Behav, 2009. **8**(8): p. 829-34.

41. Chaouloff, F., O. Berton, and P. Mormede, *Serotonin and stress.* Neuropsychopharmacology, 1999. **21**(2 Suppl): p. 28S-32S.

42. Swaab, D.F., A.M. Bao, and P.J. Lucassen, *The stress system in the human brain in depression and neurodegeneration.* Ageing Res Rev, 2005. **4**(2): p. 141-94.

43. Essex, M.J., et al, *The confluence of mental, physical, social, and academic difficulties in middle childhood. II: developing the Macarthur health and Behavior Questionnaire.* J Am Acad Child Adolesc Psychiatry, 2002. **41**(5): p. 588-603.

44. Kapoor, A., S. Petropoulos, and S.G. Matthews, *Fetal programming of hypothalamic-pituitary-adrenal (HPA) axis function and behaviour by synthetic glucocorticoids.* Brain Res Rev, 2008. **57**(2): p. 586-95.

45. Gluckman, P.D., et al, *Effect of in utero and early-life conditions on adult health and disease.* N Engl J Med, 2008. **359**(1): p. 61-73.

46. Sinclair, K.D., et al, *The developmental origins of health and disease: current theories and epigenetic mechanisms.* Soc Reprod Fertil Suppl, 2007. **64**: p. 42543.

47. Joels, M. and T.Z. Baram, *The neuro-symphony of stress.* Nat Rev Neurosci, 2009. **10**(6): p. 459-66.

48. Figueiredo, H.F., C.M. Dolgas, and J.P. Herman, *Stress activation of cortex and hippocampus is modulated by sex and stage of estrus.* Endocrinology, 2002. **143**(7): p. 2534-40.

49. McEwen, B.S., *Physiology and neurobiology of stress and adaptation: central role of the brain.* Physiol Rev, 2007. **87**(3): p. 873-904.

50. Arnsten, A.F., *Stress signalling pathways that impair prefrontal cortex structure and function.* Nat Rev Neurosci, 2009. **10**(6): p. 410-22.

51. Raymond, J.R., et al, *Multiplicity of mechanisms of serotonin receptor signal transduction.* Pharmacol Ther, 2001. **92**(2-3): p. 179-212.

52. Lupien, S.J., et al, *Effects of stress throughout the lifespan on the brain, behaviour and cognition.* Nat Rev Neurosci, 2009. **10**(6): p. 434-45.

53. McEwen, B.S., *Brain on stress: How the social environment gets under the skin.* Proc Natl Acad Sci U S A, 2012.

54. Romeo, R.D. and B.S. McEwen, *Stress and the adolescent brain.* Ann N Y Acad Sci, 2006. **1094**: p. 202-14.

55. Weiss, B., *Risk assessment: the insidious nature of neurotoxicity and the aging brain.* Neurotoxicology, 1990. **11**(2): p. 305-13.

56. Morgan, J.I. and T. Curran, *Proto-oncogenes: beyond second messengers*, in *Psychopharmacology: the forth generation of progress.* 1995, New York: Raven Press: New York. p. 631-642.

57. Elias, P.C., et al, *Hypothalamic-pituitary-adrenal axis up-regulation in rats submitted to pituitary stalk compression.* J Endocrinol, 2004. **180**(2): p. 297-302.

58. Bodnoff, S.R., et al, *Role of the central benzodiazepine receptor system in behavioural habituation to novelty.* Behav Neurosci, 1989. **103**(1): p. 209-12.

59. Dulawa, S.C. and R. Hen, *Recent advances in animal models of chronic antidepressant effects: the novelty-induced hypophagia test.* Neurosci Biobehav Rev, 2005. **29**(4-5): p. 771-83.

60. Mitsushima, D., et al, *Sex differences in the basolateral amygdala: the extracellular levels of serotonin and dopamine, and their responses to restraint stress in rats.* Eur J Neurosci, 2006. **24**(11): p. 3245-54.

61. Duchesne, A., M.M. Dufresne, and R.M. Sullivan, *Sex differences in corticolimbic dopamine and serotonin systems in the rat and the effect of postnatal handling.* Prog Neuropsychopharmacol Biol Psychiatry, 2009. **33**(2): p. 251-61.

62. Frieder, B. and V.E. Grimm, *Some long-lasting neurochemical effects of prenatal or early postnatal exposure to diazepam.* J Neurochem, 1985. **45**(1): p. 37-42.

63. Kim, M.J., et al, *The structural and functional connectivity of the amygdala: from normal emotion to pathological anxiety.* Behav Brain Res, 2011. **223**(2): p. 40310.

64. Ulrich-Lai, Y.M. and J.P. Herman, *Neural regulation of endocrine and autonomic stress responses.* Nat Rev Neurosci, 2009. **10**(6): p. 397-409.

65. Lebron-Milad, K., et al., *Sex differences in the neurobiology of fear conditioning and extinction: a preliminary fMRI study of shared sex differences with stress-arousal circuitry.* Biol Mood Anxiety Disord, 2012. **2**(1): p. 7.

66. Roozendaal, B., B.S. McEwen, and S. Chattarji, *Stress, memory and the amygdala.* Nat Rev Neurosci, 2009. **10**(6): p. 423-33.

67. Cabrera-Vera, T.M. and G. Battaglia, *Prenatal exposure to fluoxetine (Prozac) produces site-specific and age-dependent alterations in brain serotonin transporters in rat progeny: evidence from autoradiographic studies.* J Pharmacol Exp Ther, 1998. **286**(3): p. 1474-81.

68. Lesch, K.P., et al., *Association of anxiety-related traits with a polymorphism in the serotonin transporter gene regulatory region.* Science, 1996. **274**(5292): p. 1527-31.

69. Dayas, C.V., et al., *Stressor categorisation: acute physical and psychological stressors elicit distinctive recruitment patterns in the amygdala and in medullary noradrenergic cell groups.* Eur J Neurosci, 2001. **14**(7): p. 1143-52.

70. Herman, J.P., et al, *Local circuit regulation of paraventricular nucleus stress integration: glutamate-GABA connections.* Pharmacol Biochem Behav, 2002. **71**(3): p. 457-68.

71. Grzeskowiak, L.E., A.L. Gilbert, and J.L. Morrison, *Long term impact of prenatal exposure to SSRIs on growth and body weight in childhood: evidence from animal and human studies.* Reprod Toxicol, 2012. **34**(1): p. 101-9.

72. Meaney, M.J., et al., *Environmental regulation of the development of glucocorticoid receptor systems in the rat forebrain. The role of serotonin.* Ann N Y Acad Sci, 1994. **746**: p. 260-73; discussion 274, 289-93.

73. Brennan, P.A., et al, *Maternal depression and infant cortisol: influences of timing, comorbidity and treatment.* J Child Psychol Psychiatry, 2008. **49**(10): p. 1099107.

74. Oberlander, T.F., et al, *Prolonged prenatal psychotropic medication exposure alters neonatal acute pain response.* Paediatr Res, 2002. **51**(4): p. 443-53.

75. Grunau, R.E., et al, *Neonatal procedural pain exposure predicts lower cortisol and behavioural reactivity in preterm infants in the NICU.* Pain, 2005. **113**(3): p. 293300.

76. Morrison, J.L., et al, *Chronic maternal fluoxetine infusion in pregnant sheep: effects on the maternal and fetal hypothalamic-pituitary-adrenal axes.* Paediatr Res, 2004. **56**(1): p. 40-6.

77. Ishiwata, H., T. Shiga, and N. Okado, *Selective serotonin reuptake inhibitor treatment of early postnatal mice reverses their prenatal stress-induced brain dysfunction.* Neuroscience, 2005. **133**(4): p. 893-901.

78. Pawluski, J.L., et al, *Developmental fluoxetine exposure differentially alters*

central and peripheral measures of the HPA system in adolescent male and female offspring. Neuroscience, 2012. **220**: p. 131-41.

79. Viau, V. and M.J. Meaney, *Variations in the hypothalamic-pituitary-adrenal response to stress during the estrous cycle in the rat.* Endocrinology, 1991. **129**(5): p. 2503-11.

80. Kalueff, A.V., et al, *Conserved role for the serotonin transporter gene in rat and mouse neurobehavioural endophenotypes.* Neurosci Biobehav Rev, 2010. **34**(3): p. 373-86.

81. Bearer, E.L., et al, *Reward circuitry is perturbed in the absence of the serotonin transporter.* Neuroimage, 2009. **46**(4): p. 1091-104.

82. Cook, L. and J. Sepinwall, *Behavior analysis of the effects and mechanisms of action of benzodiazepines.* Psychopharmacol Bull, 1975. **11**(4): p. 53-5.

83. McAllister, B.B., V. Kiryanova, and R.H. Dyck, *Behavioural outcomes of perinatal maternal fluoxetine treatment.* Neuroscience, 2012. **226**: p. 356-66.

84. Krishnan, V. and E.J. Nestler, *The molecular neurobiology of depression.* Nature, 2008. **455**(7215): p. 894-902.

85. Laviola, G., et al, *Risk-taking behaviour in adolescent mice: psychobiological determinants and early epigenetic influence.* Neurosci Biobehav Rev, 2003. **27**(1-2): p. 19-31.

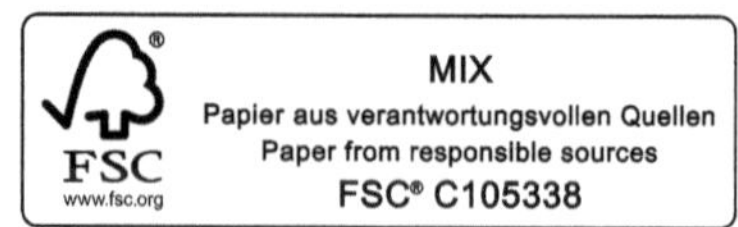

Printed by Books on Demand GmbH, Norderstedt / Germany